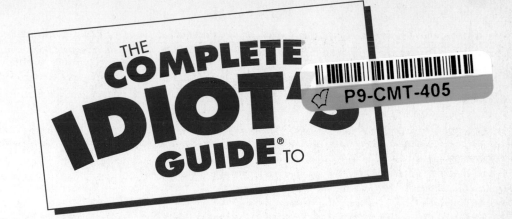

The Anti-Inflammation Diet

by Christopher P. Cannon, M.D., and
Elizabeth Vierck

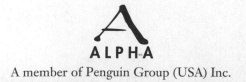

ALPHA

A member of Penguin Group (USA) Inc.

ALPHA BOOKS

Published by the Penguin Group

Penguin Group (USA) Inc., 375 Hudson Street, New York, New York 10014, U.S.A.

Penguin Group (Canada), 10 Alcorn Avenue, Toronto, Ontario, Canada M4V 3B2 (a division of Pearson Penguin Canada Inc.)

Penguin Books Ltd, 80 Strand, London WC2R 0RL, England

Penguin Ireland, 25 St Stephen's Green, Dublin 2, Ireland (a division of Penguin Books Ltd)

Penguin Group (Australia), 250 Camberwell Road, Camberwell, Victoria 3124, Australia (a division of Pearson Australia Group Pty Ltd)

Penguin Books India Pvt Ltd, 11 Community Centre, Panchsheel Park, New Delhi—110 017, India

Penguin Group (NZ), cnr Airborne and Rosedale Roads, Albany, Auckland 1310, New Zealand (a division of Pearson New Zealand Ltd)

Penguin Books (South Africa) (Pty) Ltd, 24 Sturdee Avenue, Rosebank, Johannesburg 2196, South Africa

Penguin Books Ltd, Registered Offices: 80 Strand, London WC2R 0RL, England

Publisher: *Marie Butler-Knight*
Editorial Director: *Mike Sanders*
Managing Editor: *Billy Fields*
Acquisitions Editor: *Tom Stevens*
Development Editor: *Ginny Bess Munroe*
Production Editor: *Kayla Dugger*
Copy Editor: *Amy Borrelli*
Cartoonist: *Richard King*
Cover Designer: *Bill Thomas*
Book Designers: *Trina Wurst/Kurt Owens*
Indexer: *Julie Bess*
Layout: *Ayanna Lacey*
Proofreader: *John Etchison*

Contents at a Glance

Contents

17   Exercise and Weight Control   273

Foreword

Although we all strive to be healthy, today's world has countless medical missiles that can be launched at us at any time—things like heart disease, obesity, diabetes, heart disease, and high cholesterol. While many diseases and conditions have specific treatments that can come in the form of a pill, or a needle, or a surgically guided laser, there's one prescription that serves as the foundation treatment for so many of today's frustrating and debilitating health problems: a healthy diet and exercise program.

Though many of us are so used to hinging our entire health picture on a number that's spit out from a blood test or the one that scares us on the scale, medical science has identified a critical new risk factor for heart disease and other major diseases: inflammation. It's not the kind that's associated with a swollen lip or sprained ankle, but the kind that happens *inside* your body. A natural bodily process that helps fight disease and infections, inflammation can also damage your body if it exists over a long enough time. Dr. Cannon's latest research has suggested that controlling inflammation can lead to a lower risk of heart attacks.

In *The Complete Idiot's Guide to the Anti-Inflammation Diet*, Cannon and Vierck provide a comprehensive look at inflammation—and how to reverse the effects of it. In normal language, they describe the latest medical science about inflammation, its role in many different diseases, how to test for inflammation (using, among other things, a blood test for C-reactive protein [CRP]), and what to eat to reduce it. Fortunately, medical science has recognized the importance of diet as a contributor to inflammation, and many recent studies provide reinforcement for making anti-inflammatory choices. With this book, you'll understand inflammation and its consequences, and you'll learn how to turn knowledge into action and reduce levels of inflammation in your body— by changing what you put in your mouth.

Mehmet C. Oz, M.D., is the co-author of the best-selling *You: The Owner's Manual* and is professor and vice chair of surgery and director of the Cardiovascular Institute and Complementary Medicine programs at NY Presbyterian Hospital/Columbia University.

Introduction

Inflammation is one of the hottest topics in medicine—if not the hottest topic—and with good reason. We now know the menacing role that it plays in a myriad of diseases, including heart disease. In fact, inflammation not only plays a dominant role in these diseases, it is a major risk factor itself.

Thus, treating inflammation is crucial to health. And stopping inflammation begins with eating wholesome foods.

I first discovered the importance of nutrition through the good sense of my wife, Sophie. Then a study I conducted with my colleagues at the Brigham and Women's Hospital and Harvard Medical School (and other prestigious medical centers) confirmed the key role that diet and lifestyle play in inflammation.

The study included 2,885 patients and looked at the connection between risk factors for heart disease and levels of inflammation. The results are spectacular.

We found that even when people take extensive amounts of drugs called statins (which reduce inflammation levels), diet, exercise, keeping weight down, and not smoking reduce levels even further. In fact, it is these lifestyles factors, and not the medications, that determine how low inflammation levels can actually go.

Our study showed that preventing heart disease and related inflammatory diseases is in our reach.

Obviously, we know how to get exercise and how not to smoke (although we need to overcome the barriers to actually making these lifestyle changes). Now we are fortunate because we also know what foods make inflammation worse and what foods make it better. This is a major discovery in medicine and nutrition, and the premise of the anti-inflammation diet.

We are also fortunate because, with the availability of a test called hs-CRP, we are now able to actually monitor how well the diet and other approaches are working. With this test, we draw a little of your blood and, for a relatively small price, send it to a lab for hs-CRP testing and see how high or low your inflammation levels are. This is an incredible advance in medicine, and I recommend that you and your doctor take advantage of it.

I am a cardiologist so, of course, I have come to the topic of inflammation through my research on how to prevent and treat heart disease. But, as you will see in this book, there are over a hundred diseases that are also caused by or involve inflammation, such as arthritis, Alzheimer's disease, and some types of cancer. This diet can also help stop these diseases by stopping inflammation.

Now, on to the diet. The seven principles of the anti-inflammation diet are based on the best of what we know about the science of nutrition today combined with the best of what we know about preventing inflammation. It is a science-based but practical approach to reducing the amount of inflammation in our bodies.

I also want to stress that the anti-inflammation diet is not a weight-loss diet. At the same time, when you follow these principles you are likely to achieve a healthy weight because you will be eating health-promoting foods. And, as you are about to see in the following pages, weight control is very important to reducing inflammation.

One final word: in this diet you will eat foods that taste great and are great for you. At the same time, I believe that if a diet is too strict, no one will follow it. For example, I love pasta, which is not a nutritional powerhouse. But I for one am going to enjoy pasta frequently and make accommodations in other parts of my diet. The point is to have a healthy lifestyle, reduce the risk factors for heart disease and other health conditions, and also enjoy life.

How to Use This Book

To make this book easy to use we have divided it into five areas of interest:

Part 1, "All About Inflammation," explains the key role that inflammation plays in over a hundred diseases and the connection between inflammation, diet, and other lifestyle factors. We also present the seven principles of the anti-inflammation diet.

And we give you the inside scoop on important new medical "happenings," such as hs-CRP testing to watch inflammation levels, medications that can help reduce inflammation, and the discovery that belly fat actually causes inflammation. We also include some great whole-grain recipes.

Part 2, "Diet and Inflammation," provides details on all of the seven principles of the anti-inflammation diet. They are:

1. Eat a well-balanced variety of wholesome foods.

2. Eat only unsaturated fats.

3. Eat one good source of omega-3 fatty acids every day.

4. Eat a lot of whole grains.

5. Eat healthy sources of protein.

6. Eat plenty of fruits and vegetables.

7. Eliminate refined and processed foods as much as possible.

We also cover how nutritional needs change as we grow up and grow older. And we include more recipes and lots of great tips.

Part 3, "Anti-Inflammation Guidelines for the Marketplace," helps you stay on track with the seven principles. It includes how to avoid the empty calories and bad-for-you fats that make up fast food, food-shopping strategies, and the pros and cons of supplements.

Part 4, "Exercise and Stress Reduction," provides important information on getting fit and reducing stress. We explain how to measure the intensity of activity and the importance of strength training. We also cover some of the most beneficial methods for reducing stress and learning to relax.

Part 5, "Anti-Inflammatory Cooking," discusses the most popular weight-loss diets and whether they are compatible with the seven principles of the anti-inflammation diet.

Extras

To help you get the most out of this book, we've sprinkled in some of the following helpful boxes.

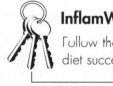

InflamWise

Follow these tips to make your diet successful.

def•i•ni•tion

Definitions relating to inflammation.

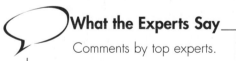

What the Experts Say

Comments by top experts.

Did You Know?

Important facts and statistics relating to inflammation and nutrition.

InflamWarnings

Important things to watch out for.

Acknowledgments

From Elizabeth Vierck:

First and foremost I would like to thank Tom Stevens at Alpha Books for his wisdom and guidance. I would also like to thank Marilyn Allen for bringing me this project and sticking through many versions of the outline and proposal.

We drew on many important data sources in the writing of this book. At the top of the list are Dr. Walter Willett, Patrick Skerret, and their colleagues at the Harvard School of Public Health. Their book, *Eat, Drink, and Be Healthy*, provides sound science-based advice that we took seriously in developing the seven principles of the anti-inflammation diet.

We also drew heavily on research conducted at or sponsored by, among others, Harvard Medical School, Brigham and Women's Hospital, Tufts University, the National Institutes of Health, the Food and Drug Administration, the National Center for Health Statistics, and the Center for Science in the Public Interest.

I would like to thank Elizabeth Yarnell for letting us print five of her delicious recipes.

Finally, I would like to personally thank my doctor, Michelle Velkoff, for taking such good care of my many inflammatory conditions for so many years. As a patient, I have been extremely lucky to have such a great doctor as a partner in my health care.

Special Thanks to the Technical Reviewer

The Complete Idiot's Guide to the Anti-Inflammation Diet was reviewed by an expert who double-checked the accuracy of what you'll learn here, to help us ensure that this book gives you everything you need to know about anti-inflammation. Special thanks are extended to Benjamin Steinberg.

Trademarks

All terms mentioned in this book that are known to be or are suspected of being trademarks or service marks have been appropriately capitalized. Alpha Books and Penguin Group (USA) Inc. cannot attest to the accuracy of this information. Use of a term in this book should not be regarded as affecting the validity of any trademark or service mark.

Part 1

All About Inflammation

If you knew you could make some changes in your life and prevent a myriad of health problems, including heart disease, stroke, diabetes, Alzheimer's disease, and arthritis, would you be up for it?

This part explains the link between disease and inflammation. And it explains how you can prevent or reduce inflammation through diet and other lifestyle factors.

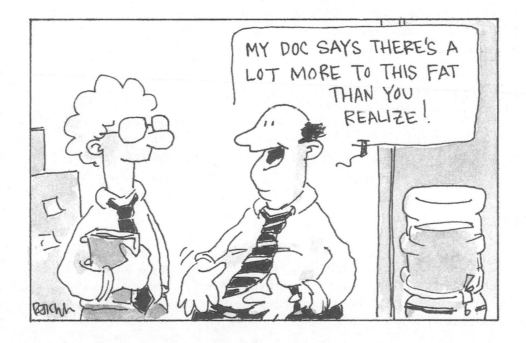

Inflammation: The Good and the Bad

In This Chapter

- Inflammation: the common thread in diseases that kill and disable
- Inflammaging
- C-reactive protein
- CRP and diet

Inflammation is now understood as a lead player in many of the diseases that can cut our lives short and make us miserable.

The good news is that if you control your inflammation by following an anti-inflammatory lifestyle, you may be able to prevent and control many health problems. You won't be preventing just heart disease. You won't be preventing just Alzheimer's disease. You won't be preventing just arthritis. (Although stopping any one of these would obviously be a very good thing.) You will be fighting all three, along with many other diseases.

In this chapter, you will learn basic information about inflammation; how it is involved in a plethora of diseases, as well as the aging process; and how to tell if you have high levels of inflammation in your body. We also cover the benefits that some medications have for reducing inflammation levels and how a healthy diet and lifestyle can reduce inflammation.

Inflammation: A Key Player in Your Body's Defense System

Under normal circumstances, *inflammation* is a protective, healing friend. It is your body's defense against attack. Simply put, if you are burned, if you cut yourself, or if a virus invades your body, fighter molecules rush in to protect you from infection. The molecules "lock down" the area of the wound to prevent contamination and focus on healing.

When the attack is over and the threat of infection is gone, inflammation is programmed by nature to depart and be ready to defend any new attacks. However, sometimes this programming crashes and inflammation does not leave, leading to a long-lasting condition that festers away quietly.

def•i•ni•tion

Inflammation is the body's reaction to injury or to other irritations and stresses such as infections, allergies, chemical irritations, and sometimes loss of function. Common reactions are pain, swelling, redness, and heat. Any area of the body may become inflamed.

Constant attacks on your body by too many saturated fats, too much body fat, smoking, and other assaults can also lead to long-lasting inflammation—a condition called silent, low-grade, or chronic inflammation.

Silent inflammation can invade with no known cause or "trigger." It's sneaky. It can fall below the pain threshold so victims do not even notice it. This type of inflammation has been the subject of a great deal of research in recent years because of its connection to so many health problems.

The Common Thread

Inflammation is the common thread that runs through many diseases. Some of these health conditions are fatal. Many are incapacitating. We provide details on these inflammation-related diseases in Chapter 2. However, here is a brief overview of them:

◆ The three top killers in the United States: heart disease, cancer, and stroke

◆ Diabetes

◆ Alzheimer's disease

◆ Many of the numerous forms of arthritis including rheumatoid arthritis and lupus

◆ Inflammatory bowel disease (ulcerative colitis and Crohn's disease)

◆ Age-related macular degeneration

◆ Sepsis (infection in the bloodstream)

◆ Other autoimmune diseases, including lupus and multiple sclerosis

◆ Hundreds of diseases ending in *itis*, such as meningitis

◆ Acne

◆ Allergies

def•i•ni•tion

Itis is a suffix that is used in medical terms to describe an inflammatory disease. When you see it at the end of a word it means "inflammation of." For example, *colitis* means inflammation of the colon and *pancreatitis* means inflammation of the pancreas.

Inflammation's symptoms differ according to the part of the body that is under attack. For example, your blood vessels can develop atherosclerosis as a result of inflammation. In this case the first symptom you recognize might be a heart attack. Or you might fall and twist your ankle, which immediately hurts, turns red, and swells. Or, you might develop macular degeneration and your first symptom is, tragically, loss of vision.

Inflammation and Aging

Recent research shows that what most of us think of as the inevitable forces of aging—such as the wasting away of muscle, wrinkling skin, and the high risk of acute and chronic disease—is really due to inflammation. In fact, if you can reduce inflammation you can also reduce the risk of or delay many of these "effects of aging."

Noted Italian researcher Claudio Franceschi believes so strongly in the aging-is-inflammation connection that he calls the process "inflammaging." According to Franceschi, "Inflammaging is the common and most important driving force of age-related disease."

The inflammaging idea has been championed by Dr. Caleb Finch, director of the University of Southern California Alzheimer's Disease Research Center. Finch says that a major reason why people lived longer in the last century than ever before is because they were exposed "to fewer infectious diseases and other sources of inflammation."

Inflammaging has also gotten the public's attention through the writings and appearances of the popular doctor Andrew Weil. In fact, Weil's prescription for reducing aging-related health problems is to follow an anti-inflammatory diet.

Inflammation and C-Reactive Protein (CRP)

How do you know if you have high levels of inflammation in your body? There is an inexpensive blood test that can help you and your doctor determine your levels of inflammation.

def•i•ni•tion

C-reactive protein (CRP) is a protein in the blood whose level rises dramatically during inflammatory processes occurring in the body. It is also believed to play a role as an early defense system against infections.

If any part of you is inflamed, the *C-reactive protein (CRP)* levels in your blood will be high. As inflammation increases, your CRP level also increases.

CRP measurement is not new. Doctors have used it for decades to follow and monitor the care of patients with lupus, rheumatoid arthritis, and other inflammatory conditions.

Many studies have now shown an association between high CRP levels and heart disease. This is the case even for people with normal cholesterol levels!

Where Does CRP Come From?

CRP is produced by the liver, fat around the stomach area, and within the two arteries that supply blood to the heart (called coronary arteries or vessels).

InflamWarnings

If, according to blood tests, your cholesterol level is low or normal (below 200 mg/dl), do not assume that you are low risk for heart disease. If your CRP levels are high, regardless of your cholesterol reading, you are high risk for cardiovascular problems, such as heart attacks or strokes.

The amount of CRP that bodies produce varies from person to person, depending on genetic history and lifestyle. If you smoke, have high blood pressure, are overweight, and don't exercise, your levels are likely to be high. If you are lean and athletic, there is a good chance your CRP levels are low.

CRP and Risk Factors for Heart Disease

The American Heart Association warns that if your CRP levels are high, and you have a condition called unstable angina (an increasing or "crescendo" pattern of chest pain that occurs with little activity) or a prior heart attack, you are high risk for a heart attack. Furthermore, if you would have a heart attack with these risk factors, your chance of surviving it is much lower.

Researchers have recently also identified the following risk factors that, if coupled with high CRP levels, spell trouble:

◆ If you have high blood pressure and a high CRP level, you are at much greater risk of a heart attack or stroke.

◆ The risk of high blood pressure is high if your CRP level is high.

◆ If you have high levels of both CRP and LDL (the bad cholesterol), you are very high risk for heart attack or stroke.

◆ If you have diabetes and high CRP levels, you have a high risk of having a future heart attack or stroke.

◆ If you have had a medical procedure to open up your arteries (balloon angio-plasty) and your CRP levels are high, there is a risk that the arteries will close back up.

These facts emphasize the importance of following an anti-inflammatory diet and life-style, which we introduce later in this chapter.

CRP Testing

Changes in CRP levels are often the first sign of inflammation or infection in the body. In fact, your CRP level may rise even before you feel pain.

> ### Did You Know?
>
> A study published in the *New England Journal of Medicine* concluded that C-reactive protein predicted heart attacks and strokes better than any other laboratory test.

> ### InflamWise
>
> CRP testing can fluctuate widely. If your hs-CRP level is above 10mg/l, you should have the test repeated after 2 to 3 weeks, as the high level may be from an infection and not due to an underlying disease with inflammation.

To measure your C-reactive protein level, your doctor will draw your blood and order a "high-sensitivity" CRP or hs-CRP test from the laboratory. hs-CRP levels are measured by milligrams per liter, written as (mg/l). CRP testing costs between $12 and $16. They also require only a small amount of blood.

The Centers for Disease Control and American Heart Association developed a widely used classification system of hs-CRP to determine risk for heart disease:

- Low risk—less than 1 milligram per liter of blood
- Moderate risk—1 to 3 milligrams per liter
- High risk—over 3 milligrams per liter

A higher or increasing amount of C-reactive protein in your blood suggests raging inflammation.

This system might change with more research, but at this writing it is the medical standard.

At What Age?

The best time to start getting your CRP levels tested is now—regardless of your age. If you are in your teens or 20s, your current CRP level will provide a comparison for your levels later in life.

Medicine and Inflammation

Four categories of medications can help ease inflammation. They are statins, NSAIDS, anti-diabetes drugs, and steroids.

Statins and CRP

Dr. Christopher Cannon, lead author of this book, has done extensive research on drugs used to treat people at risk for heart disease. The drugs, called statins, stop your body from making too much cholesterol and increase your liver's ability to remove it from your blood. They also slightly raise high-density lipoprotein (HDL), which is good for your heart.

Did You Know?
Here are some facts about CRP: ◆ About one quarter of Americans have an hs-CRP level above 3mg/l, placing them in a high-risk group for heart disease. Studies have found that the risk for heart attack in people in the upper third of CRP levels is *twice* that of those whose levels are in the lower third.   ◆ Most infections are associated with CRP levels above 10mg/dl.   ◆ People with autoimmune diseases (such as rheumatoid arthritis or lupus or cancer) often have elevated CRP levels.   ◆ CRP levels are higher in people who are obese.

An interesting new discovery is that statins, usually prescribed to lower cholesterol, also reduce CRP. (Cholesterol, of course, is a fatlike substance in your body and in many foods. Everyone needs some cholesterol in their blood, but too much of it can cause heart disease.)

We are lucky that we have these drugs available to us. They are saving lives. Ask your doctor if a statin drug is appropriate for you. However, remember that the best medicine is prevention, beginning with following an anti-inflammatory diet and lifestyle.

NSAIDs (Non-Steroidal Anti-Inflammatory Drugs)

In the last decade or so a flurry of research has shown that NSAIDs (non-steroidal anti-inflammatory drugs), such as aspirin and Aleve®, help control many inflammatory diseases, including heart disease, arthritis, and even Alzheimer's disease.

In short, people who take NSAIDs, such as the miracle everyday drug aspirin, appear to have less inflammation-related disease than people who do not take them. However, side effects can occur, such as bleeding. Your doctor might consider NSAIDS to reduce inflammation in some situations.

Steroids and CRP

A third category of drugs that can ease inflammation is corticosteroids, man-made drugs that closely resemble a hormone called cortisol that your body produces naturally. Corticosteroids are often referred to by the shortened term "steroids." They are not the same as the hormone-related steroids that some athletes use.

Common steroid medicines include cortisone, prednisone, and methylprednisolone. Prednisone is commonly used to treat some types of arthritis.

Steroids can have unpleasant side effects and are used only when there are no other options. Some common problems are: increased appetite, weight gain, sudden mood swings, muscle weakness, blurred vision, increased growth of body hair, bruising easily, low resistance to infection, swollen or "puffy" face, osteoporosis (bone-weakening disease), worsening of diabetes, high blood pressure, stomach irritation, nervousness, restlessness, sleeping difficulties, cataracts or glaucoma, water retention, or swelling.

InflamWarnings

Some people are allergic to aspirin and other NSAIDs, which can cause the serious breathing disease asthma.

The first symptoms are a runny nose, sneezing, and facial flushing. You can develop an aspirin allergy even if you have taken them in the past and had no problems. If you take aspirin and have had any of these symptoms, check with your doctor.

Diabetes Drugs and CRP

If you are diabetic, here is some good news: relatively recent studies have shown that the diabetes drugs Actos and Avandia, known as TZDs or thiazolidinediones, may help fight inflammation. They are particularly effective in reducing CRP levels when taken with statins.

How to Reduce CRP

The following sections provide key information on how you can reduce your CRP levels.

You Are in Control

In the introduction to this book, Dr. Cannon wrote about the startling results of the study he and his colleagues at Harvard Medical School (and other prestigious medical centers) conducted. The study showed that even when people take high dosages of drugs that lower CRP levels, diet and other lifestyle factors determine how low they can actually go.

According to Dr. Cannon, "Because of the results of this study and others, there is a new standard of care emerging in medicine to check CRP levels to see how patients are doing health-wise. I call this testing the *global risk barometer*. With this one measure—CRP—you can find out if you are high risk for getting a number of diseases. And, if you are, it is clear what you can do about it."

Here is the bottom line: because of CRP testing and the knowledge base that Dr. Cannon and his colleagues have built, the future is bright. You can control a major "driver" behind heart disease, stroke, Alzheimer's disease, and other illnesses. Have your CRP levels tested regularly and, if they are not normal, step up the anti-inflammatory practices we describe in this book. The ball is in your court.

def•i•ni•tion

Global risk barometer is using CRP testing on a regular basis to measure health. If your CRP levels are not normal, it means that you should work to reduce them by following the anti-inflammation diet and lifestyle.

The CRP/Diet Connection

Hippocrates, the father of Western medicine, said, "Let your food be your medicine, and your medicine be your food." There is clear evidence that a healthful diet is great medicine for inflammation. It involves eating nutrient-rich foods and eliminating empty calories.

The anti-inflammation diet has seven principles:

1. Eat a well-balanced variety of wholesome foods.

2. Eat only unsaturated fats.

3. Eat one good source of omega-3 fatty acids every day.

4. Eat a lot of whole grains.

5. Eat lean sources of protein.

6. Eat plenty of fruits and vegetables.

7. Eliminate processed and refined foods as much as possible.

In addition, to reduce inflammation and enhance the positive impact of the anti-inflammation diet, it is important to also follow an anti-inflammatory lifestyle—get regular exercise, keep your weight in control, and reduce the stresses in your life.

The point of the anti-inflammation diet is to eat foods that taste great and are great for you. You will, by eating a lot of fresh foods. Eat whole grains, not refined rice or food made with refined flour. Choose lean meats and eat them only for special occasions. Eat lots of the good-for-you type of fish. Make olive oil, walnuts, and other nuts your sources of fat. Cut out butter; cut out margarine. Cut out processed foods as much as you possibly can. Have a little wine (unless drinking alcohol is a problem for you).

The anti-inflammation diet isn't a diet specifically to lose weight. It is not low carb, low fat, low calorie, or highly regimented. It is an approach to the way we eat to reduce the amount of inflammation in our bodies. It is a way of life.

However, a word of caution: if you are overweight, you are putting your body under tremendous stress. Body fat is a direct cause of inflammation. People who are overweight store high levels of arachidonic acid (AA), the building blocks of pro-inflammatory cells called eicosanoids. And body fat makes C-reactive protein.

A word of encouragement: after you start eating a healthful diet, you will probably lose weight if you also exercise and do not overeat. We cover more about the effects of being overweight on inflammation in Chapter 3.

The Mediterranean Connection

For over four decades the typical Mediterranean diet has gotten good press. Hundreds of books have been written about it. A current popular diet called the Sonoma Diet is based on it.

Along with a couple of refinements, the Mediterranean diet fits the description of a healthful, anti-inflammatory diet. The traditional diets of the Mediterranean region consisted of foods from a rich diversity of sun-drenched plants. They ate lots of fruits, vegetables, whole grains, beans, nuts, and seeds. Olive oil was the area's principle source of fat. Fish and meats were served only on special occasions.

These were the old ways of people whose countries border the Mediterranean Sea.

The benefits of the traditional Mediterranean diet first gained attention in the early 1960s, when physician Ancel Keys brought together a group of scientists to look at disease and the diet patterns of seven countries. Their conclusion was that the Mediterranean-style diet was responsible for the generally good health and lack of disease of people living in countries bordering the Mediterranean Sea, such as

Greece, Crete, and southern Italy, in comparison to people living away from the Mediterranean. People from the Mediterranean area were particularly heart healthy.

Keys began following the Mediterranean diet in the 1950s and wrote a cookbook to promote it. He died in 2004, a month before his 101st birthday. Whether his long life was a result of his diet, good genes, or both, he is known for promoting healthful nutrition instead of, as he put it, "the North American habit for making the stomach the garbage disposal for a long list of harmful foods."

A plethora of recent evidence has confirmed and expanded on Keys's study. One of the researchers studying the Mediterranean diet is Dr. Demosthenes Panagiotakos of the University of Athens in Greece. He says, "The Mediterranean diet, independent of any other factor, reduces levels of inflammation."

The doctor's comments are based on a research project called the Attica Study. He and his colleagues studied the dietary habits of 2,282 men and women, aged 18 to 89 years, who had no history or signs of heart disease. The more participants who followed the Mediterranean diet, the better their CRP levels.

Another study found that the Mediterranean diet, along with exercise three times a week for 3 months, caused CRP levels in 65 heart disease patients to drop by almost a third (31 percent). In addition, their body fat was reduced by an average of 5 percent and their exercise capacity improved 36 percent. This is just some of the recent research that has shown the benefits of following a healthful diet and lifestyle.

Our philosophy toward eating to prevent inflammation is a refinement of the Mediterranean diet. The nutritional approach that we believe works best was developed by Dr. Walter Willett and his colleagues. Dr. Willett is professor of epidemiology and nutrition at Harvard Medical School. He draws on the most up-to-date research in nutrition and also emphasizes exercise and taking a multivitamin every day. Dr. Willett's diet, which he calls the Healthy Eating Pyramid, incorporates and expands on the Mediterranean diet. To learn more about the diet, see Chapter 4.

What, Me Worry?

Let's look back for a minute to see what we've discussed so far. Because it is the nation's biggest killer, we covered a lot of information about inflammation in relation to heart disease. As we also mentioned, inflammation plays a key role in many other diseases that can kill or incapacitate.

We also established that inflammation can be measured by testing CRP levels in the blood. And we've discussed how a healthful diet and lifestyle can reduce inflammation and CRP levels in your body.

At this point many people say, "Yeah, but …"

"Yeah, but I walk the golf course a couple of times a week, I'm okay."

"Yeah, but we're all going to die of something, and I don't want to give up my morning muffin and coffee with cream."

"Yeah, but inflammation is an old person's problem. I'm only in my 30s."

Well, if you live longer and are healthier you can play more golf. That daily muffin and coffee with cream may be adding to your morning aches and pains. And the researcher Francesci has proven that inflammation when young leads to age-related problems later in life. You're never too young to start living healthfully.

It is never too early, never too late to use the principles in this book and learn how to defeat inflammation.

Ancel Keys' Recipes

Ancel Keys and his wife, Margaret, popularized dried beans in the American diet. Their cookbook, *The Benevolent Bean*, was a bestseller in the 1960s. The following recipes are updated and based on the Keys' famous book (Noondays Press, 1967).

Balkan Bean Soup

1 lb. (2½ cups) dried white beans

2 stalks celery, chopped

¼ cup tomato purée

2 large onions, chopped

2 large carrots, chopped

2 TB. minced parsley

¼ cup olive oil

Salt and pepper to taste

Wash beans and soak overnight in 3 quarts of water or use the microwave method: put washed beans in a 5-quart glass container with 8 cups of water. Cover with an all-glass lid or plastic wrap, then cook at full power for 8 to 10 minutes or until boiling. Let stand for 1 hour or longer, stirring occasionally, then drain.

Put all ingredients in a pot and cook until beans are soft but still whole (2 hours or longer).

Squash and Bean Soup

1 lb. dried white beans

2 lbs. hubbard, buttercup, or other hard yellow squash, peeled and cubed

2 TB. olive oil

1 pint skim or low-fat milk

Salt and pepper to taste

Soak and simmer beans as described in previous recipe. Drain beans and reserve liquid. Cook squash in oil in covered pan over low heat. Drain beans, reserving liquid. Purée both beans and squash in a blender or food processor and add to bean liquor. Add milk, season with salt and pepper, and serve hot.

The Least You Need to Know

◆ Inflammation is directly linked to heart disease, as well as nearly a hundred other diseases, including arthritis, Alzheimer's, and diabetes.

◆ Many common signs of aging are actually caused by inflammation.

◆ Have your CRP levels tested now so that you can use your current level as a baseline for future, regular tests.

◆ Work with your doctor to treat inflammation that is out of control.

◆ Remember if your doctor has prescribed statins, NSAIDs, steroids, or TZDs for you, they may also lower inflammation.

◆ Follow an anti-inflammatory diet to prevent and control numerous diseases.

Chapter 2

When Inflammation Is Out of Control

In This Chapter

- ◆ Inflammation's role in the top three killers—heart disease, cancer, and stroke
- ◆ How inflammation causes heart attacks
- ◆ How inflammation may cause Alzheimer's disease
- ◆ Inflammation's role in many other common diseases including diabetes, inflammatory digestive disease, and acne
- ◆ Common forms of arthritis and how they are related to inflammation
- ◆ The hundreds of diseases that are named for their inflammatory states such as colitis and vasculitis

From your toes to your brain, inflammation is associated with or a part of many illnesses. It can also rage out of control and actually cause serious disease. In fact, inflammation is involved in many of the diseases that eventually kill us or cause serious disability, such as heart disease, stroke, cancer, diabetes, and Alzheimer's disease.

In this chapter, you will learn about the broad range of diseases associated with inflammation—those that are life-threatening and those that are milder but can result in chronic health problems.

The following table lists the prevalence of some common inflammatory diseases.

Number of People with Inflammatory Diseases in the United States

Hay fever	27.2 million
Asthma	20 million
Cardiovascular diseases	71 million
Arthritis (all types combined)	49 million
Osteoarthritis	21 million
Rheumatoid arthritis	2.1 million
Alzheimer's disease	4.5 million
Gum disease	5.6 million

Just glancing at this chapter should give you plenty of incentive to practice the anti-inflammatory diet, which can help keep these diseases away or, if they occur, help control them.

Heart Disease: The Top Killer in the United States

When death comes it is usually the result of heart disease, which is the clogging of the blood vessels to and from your heart. Inflammation plays a central role in this disease, the top killer of both men and women.

Did You Know?

Your arteries are the blood vessels that carry oxygen-rich blood to tissues in your body. Plaques, which are deposits of fatty material, can build up within artery walls. Inflammatory reactions within the deposits of plaques on the innermost layer of the walls of arteries are known as atherosclerotic plaques. These plaques can cause blood clots and narrowed arteries, a condition known as atherosclerosis, which can lead to a heart attack or other life-threatening problems.

High levels of CRP have been found in atherosclerosis, the hardware behind heart disease. According to the American Heart Association, the higher your CRP levels, the higher your risk of developing heart attack or stroke.

You may hear your doctor refer to CRP as an inflammatory "marker." Today most doctors order a *high-sensitivity CRP* test if they suspect their patient has heart disease or other inflammation-related problems. The test measures the amount of inflammation you have in your body.

def•i•ni•tion

High-sensitivity CRP is a test that measures the amount of a certain protein in the blood, which can indicate acute inflammation.

How Does Inflammation Cause Heart Attacks?

Scientists and the media used to use a clogged plumbing analogy to describe the process that leads to atherosclerosis. The idea was that LDL cholesterol (the bad cholesterol) clogged the pipes, which shut off blood flow. Today scientists have developed a new picture of the disease.

Blood vessels are narrow tubes of layered, living tissue. LDL cholesterol doesn't just lodge in arterial walls—it damages them. The injury stirs up inflammation. Legions of protective cells come to the rescue. (That's inflammation's job, after all.)

While the protective cells do their work they make a mess, enlarging and changing deposits of LDL cholesterol into plaques (deposits of fatty material). Other inflammatory molecules weaken the cap on top of the plaque. Eventually the cap bursts. The contents of the plaque make another mess. Clotting factors in the blood come "to the rescue." The result is a massive blood clot, a blocked artery, and a heart attack or stroke.

Did You Know?

The lifetime risk for heart disease is two in three for men and more than one in two for women.

—Source: *Heart Disease and Stroke Statistics—2006 Update* (American Heart Association, 2005)

Signs of Heart Disease

Some of the earliest recognizable signs of heart disease are chest pain (angina); squeezing, fullness, or pain in the center of the chest; and/or pain in the shoulders, neck, or arms. Women may also have nontypical symptoms such as stomach upset, dizziness, rapid heartbeats, shortness of breath, and fatigue. Heart disease is sometimes sneaky. Some people will have none of these symptoms; others will have many of them.

It is crucial that you immediately call 911 if any of these symptoms come on quickly for you or a loved one. And research has found that chewing one regular strength adult aspirin right away when you notice symptoms can help lessen damage to your heart. It helps prevent blood clotting.

Cancer: The Second Top Killer in the United States

Although heart attacks are the leading cause of death today, for most of us, our greatest health fear is the "big C"—*cancer*. The most common cancers, while occurring in different areas of the body with different cell "signatures," all have something in common—inflammation. Breast, cervical, ovarian, liver, esophagus, stomach, colon, urinary bladder, and pancreatic cancers all have links to inflammation.

def•i•ni•tion

Cancer is the general name for hundreds of diseases in which some of the body's cells become abnormal and divide without control. Cancer cells may invade nearby tissues and spread to other parts of the body (metastasize).

New research has shown that most precancerous and cancerous cells show signs of inflammation. And there is evidence that the longer inflammation is present, the higher the risk of getting an associated cancer. For example, people with inflammatory bowel disease (UC or Crohn's) have a five- to seven-fold increase in their risk for developing colon cancer.

What the Experts Say

Sometimes inflammation directly causes cancer, like the match that starts the fire. In other cases, inflammation causes an already established cancer to grow and spread, which is more like pouring gasoline on cancer's flame.
—William Joel Meggs, M.D., Ph.D.

Stroke: The Number-Three Killer in the United States

The inflammation that is part of heart disease can also cause strokes due to a blood clot or bleeding suddenly stopping the flow of blood to the brain. Sometimes called brain attacks, strokes occur when brain cells are deprived of blood and they stop functioning. If the loss of blood lasts too long, brain cells die.

The warning signs of stroke are:

◆ Sudden numbness or weakness of the face, arm, or leg, especially on one side of the body

◆ Sudden confusion, trouble speaking or understanding

◆ Sudden trouble seeing in one or both eyes

◆ Sudden trouble walking, dizziness, loss of balance or coordination

◆ Sudden, severe headache with no known cause

Diabetes

Inflammation of the blood vessels, which we know increases the risk of heart disease and stroke, is also a strong predictor of Type II diabetes. In one study, women who had inflamed blood vessels were five times as likely to develop diabetes as other women.

Did You Know?

Many people have referred to a recent rise in diabetes as an epidemic. Here are some statistics from the Centers for Disease Control and Prevention that back up this claim:

◆ More than 17 million Americans have diabetes.

◆ In the United States diabetes has increased nearly 50 percent in the past 10 years alone.

◆ One in three Americans born in 2000 will develop diabetes.

Diabetes, the number-six killer in the United States, is a disease in which damaging amounts of sugar build up in the blood. The buildup is caused by the body not being able to use (Type I) or produce (Type II) *insulin*, which it needs to convert food into energy. Being overweight is a major risk factor for Type II diabetes.

Almost all of the problems diabetics develop, which can be serious and life-threatening, are the result of damage of blood vessels. Diabetes can lead to blindness, loss of toes and limbs, nerve damage, and diseases of the heart, eyes, and kidneys.

def•i•ni•tion

Insulin is a hormone that is needed to convert sugar, starches, and other food into energy.

Inflammatory Bowel Disease

The effects of inflammation-related digestive problems can range from that uncomfortable feeling you get about an hour after you polish off Aunt May's lasagna to painful and serious conditions such as Crohn's disease.

The digestive (or gastrointestinal [GI]) tract includes the esophagus, stomach, small intestine, large intestine (colon), rectum, and anus. A number of conditions in the tract involve inflammation, including:

◆ Inflammatory bowel disease (IBD), the general name for diseases that cause inflammation in the intestines.

◆ Ulcerative colitis, inflammation and sores (ulcers) in the lining of the large intestine.

◆ Esophagitis, inflammation of the esophagus, the hollow tube that leads from the throat to the stomach.

◆ Inflammation in the rectum and lower part of the colon.

◆ Bleeding from the colon.

◆ Bloody diarrhea.

Alzheimer's Disease

Alzheimer's disease is a progressive brain disease that gradually destroys a person's memory and ability to learn, reason, make judgments, communicate, and carry out daily activities.

Alzheimer's disease is not a normal part of aging. It is a devastating, heartbreaking disorder of the brain.

As Alzheimer's progresses, victims' personality and behavior change, and they become anxious, suspicious, or agitated. They also have delusions or hallucinations. Eventually, they will need complete care. If the victim has no other serious illness, the loss of brain function itself causes death.

Although there is currently no cure for Alzheimer's, new treatments are on the horizon.

The following are the top 10 warning signs of Alzheimer's disease:

- Memory loss that affects day-to-day function
- Difficulty performing familiar tasks
- Problems with language
- Disorientation of time and place
- Poor or decreased judgment
- Problems with abstract thinking
- Misplacing things
- Changes in mood and behavior
- Changes in personality
- Loss of initiative

Based on their ground-breaking research, a group of scientists at the Scripps Research Institute in California have proposed a new theory about the cause of Alzheimer's disease. They believe that inflammation is the switch that turns on the disease.

According to the researchers, inflammation makes abnormal substances out of normal building blocks of cells (molecules). These abnormal substances then change certain proteins in the brain (amyloid beta proteins) and cause them to misfold. These misfolded proteins are thought to be a major player in Alzheimer's disease.

Did You Know?

The following are notable facts about Alzheimer's disease:

◆ An estimated 4.5 million Americans have Alzheimer's disease.

◆ By 2050 the number of people with Alzheimer's could reach 16 million.

◆ One in ten Americans say they have a family member with Alzheimer's and one in three know someone with the disease.

◆ Increasing age is the greatest risk factor for Alzheimer's. One in ten individuals over 65 and nearly half of those over 85 are affected. Rare, inherited forms of Alzheimer's disease can strike individuals as early as their 30s and 40s.

—Source: Alzheimer's Association

Arthritis

The hallmark of arthritis is inflammation. The word "arthritis" literally means "inflammation of the joint." There are more than 100 types of the disease, many of which are caused by inflammation going awry and attacking its own cells.

When inflammation strikes joints, increased numbers of cells and inflammatory substances cause irritation and wear away cartilage (the cushions at the ends of the bones). This process causes swelling. Flulike symptoms can accompany the inflammation.

The inflammation that accompanies arthritis can affect your heart and other body organs. The symptoms depend on the particular organ affected. For example, inflammation of the heart (myocarditis) can cause shortness of breath and fluid retention. Inflammation of the small tubes that transport air to the lungs may cause asthma attacks. And inflammation of the kidneys (nephritis) may lead to high blood pressure and/or kidney failure.

The following sections cover the major types of arthritis and their connections to inflammation.

Osteoarthritis (OA)

The most common type of arthritis is osteoarthritis. However, the role of inflammation in the disease is controversial. Studies of cells show that there is inflammation in joints damaged by osteoarthritis, but not as much as in other types of arthritis, such as rheumatoid arthritis.

Stiffness, joint pain, and swelling are the earliest symptoms of OA. In contrast to inflammatory arthritis, activity or weight-bearing activity can make osteoarthritis painful. However, as luck would have it, people with osteoarthritis must exercise regularly to keep the joints lubricated and muscles strong.

> **Did You Know?**
>
> Osteoarthritis is the most prevalent form of arthritis. It affects 70 percent of adults between 55 and 78 years old.
> —Source: Cleveland Clinic

Rheumatoid Arthritis (RA)

Rheumatoid arthritis is one of the most common and serious forms of arthritis. It is caused by inflammation of the membrane lining the joint, called the synovium, which leads to pain, stiffness, warmth, redness, and swelling. The inflamed synovium can invade and damage bone and cartilage, causing joint deformities, loss of movement, and limitation of activities. According to the Mayo Clinic's Dr. Maradit Kremers, "We believe that inflammation is a strong risk factor for cardiovascular disease among rheumatoid arthritis patients."

RA can start at any age, including during childhood. It affects two to three times more women than men.

Gout

Gout causes sudden, severe attacks of pain and tenderness, redness, warmth, and swelling in some joints. It is the result of a buildup in the body of too much uric acid, which forms crystals in the joints and causes inflammation. (Uric acid is a substance that normally forms when the body breaks down waste products called purines.)

The disease can be inherited or happen as a complication of another condition.

Gout usually affects one joint at a time—often the big toe. Episodes develop quickly. The first time it strikes is usually at night.

Gout can be caused by:

◆ Drinking too much alcohol

◆ Eating and drinking too much of certain foods and liquids

◆ Surgery

> **Did You Know?**
>
> If you have gout, stay away from beer and other alcoholic beverages; anchovies, sardines in oil, fish roes, and herring; yeast; red meat; organ meats (liver, kidneys, and sweetbreads); legumes (dried beans and peas); meat extracts, consommé, and gravies; and mushrooms, spinach, asparagus, and cauliflower.

- Sudden, severe illness

- Crash diets

- Joint injury

- Chemotherapy

If you are a male over age 40 you are the most at risk for gout, but it can affect anyone of any age. Women with gout usually develop it after menopause.

Polymyalgia Rheumatica (PMR)

Polymyalgia rheumatica is a common cause of aching and stiffness in older adults. Symptoms are worse at night and when getting out of bed in the morning.

PMR can be difficult to diagnose because it rarely causes swollen joints or other abnormalities. The symptoms of PMR are aching and stiffness about the upper arms, neck, thighs, and buttocks. Low doses of corticosteroids usually greatly relieve symptoms.

Nothing to Sneeze At: Allergies

def•i•ni•tion

Asthma is an inflammatory lung disorder in which the airways become obstructed. It can cause death if not treated.

If you have allergies, your body overreacts to things (triggers) that usually cause no reaction in other people. Triggers vary. You may be allergic to dogs and not cats. Your best friend may be allergic to cats and not dogs.

Symptoms of allergies are inflammation, sneezing, wheezing, coughing, and itching. Many allergies are linked to serious inflammatory illnesses, such as the breathing disorder *asthma*.

Acne

Acne is an inflammatory disorder of the skin's oil glands and the areas where hair grows. It is best known for its characteristic "zits," pimples, and deep pustules (small, inflamed, pus-filled, blisterlike lesions).

Acne begins when oil and dead skin cells get trapped in pores in the skin. It affects about 80 percent of people between the ages of 12 and 24, but adults can get it also. If severe enough, acne can leave permanent scars.

Despite what your mom might have said, acne does not come from chocolate, french fries, or dirty skin. However, following the anti-inflammation diet and washing your face well enough to keep your pores clean can help prevent and control acne.

Age-Related Macular Degeneration

Age-related macular degeneration (AMD) has the unhappy distinction of being the leading cause of blindness in people over 55 in the United States. Age-related macular degeneration is an eye disease that affects the macula, a part of the retina that allows you to see fine detail.

What the Experts Say

There is growing evidence that chronic inflammation plays a role in the development of macular degeneration.

—Joan W. Miller, M.D., chairwoman, Department of Ophthalmology, Harvard University

Most vision loss in age-related macular degeneration is caused by the growth of abnormal blood vessels under the retina. With it, the vessels bleed and scar tissue is formed, blocking vision. One phase in the growth of these blood vessels involves inflammation.

Degeneration of the macula causes blurred central vision or a blind spot in the center of your visual field.

def•i•ni•tion

Degeneration is the deterioration of specific tissues, cells, or organs with impairment or loss of function.

Other Autoimmune Diseases

In autoimmune diseases, the body's immune system, which normally fights such things as bee stings and viruses, does not shut off after the trigger is gone. Instead the immune system attacks the body's own healthy tissue, causing more inflammation and destroying tissue. In other words, the body attacks itself. The numerous forms of arthritis described previously are examples of common autoimmune diseases.

Any disease in which *cytotoxic* cells attack the body's own tissues is considered an autoimmune problem. Because autoimmunity can affect any organ in the body (including brain, skin, kidney, lungs, liver, heart, and thyroid), the symptoms of the disease depend upon the site affected. Autoimmune diseases include, but are not limited to:

def•i•ni•tion

Cytotoxic means of or relating to substances that are poisonous to cells.

What the Experts Say

Whatever the ultimate cause, the damage caused by autoimmunity has an obvious immediate cause: inappropriate, unchecked inflammation.

—Andrew Weil, M.D., founder and director of the Program in Integrative Medicine (PIM) at the University of Arizona, and author of numerous books, including *Healthy Aging*

Did You Know?

Approximately 20 percent of the population has autoimmune diseases. Women are more likely than men to be affected.

—American Autoimmune and Related Diseases Association

- ◆ Allergies (see text earlier in this chapter).

- ◆ Celiac disease, an inability to tolerate wheat protein. Symptoms include foul-smelling diarrhea and emaciation, often accompanied by lactose intolerance.

- ◆ Crohn's disease, a serious inflammation of the small intestine causing frequent bouts of diarrhea, abdominal pain, nausea, fever, and weight loss.

- ◆ Hashimoto's thyroiditis, a disease of the thyroid gland, resulting in its enlargement (goiter).

- ◆ Multiple sclerosis (MS), a long-term degenerative disease of the central nervous system, leading to muscular weakness, loss of coordination, and speech and visual disturbances.

- ◆ Hormone-related (endocrine) disorders in the same family as Hashimoto's thyroiditis, including Type I diabetes mellitus, Graves' disease, and Addison's disease.

- ◆ Sjogren's Syndrome, a chronic disease in which white blood cells attack the moisture-producing glands. The hallmark symptoms are dry eyes and dry mouth, but it can affect many organs and cause fatigue.

- ◆ Systemic Lupus Erythematosus, a chronic rheumatic disease that affects joints, muscles, and other parts of the body.

The "Itises"

"Itis" is a Greek term that means inflammation. For example, *colitis* is literally "inflammation of the colon."

Any area of your body can become inflamed. There are literally hundreds of medical terms that end in "-itis" and describe inflammatory conditions. The following list will give you an idea of how prevalent these diseases are in our society:

◆ Appendicitis, inflammation of the appendix, a closed-ended, narrow tube that attaches to the colon. Inflammation and infection spread through the wall of the appendix, which can rupture. After rupture, infection can spread throughout the stomach area.

◆ Arthritis (described earlier in this chapter).

◆ Bronchitis, a condition that occurs when the inner walls that line the main air passageways of your lungs become infected and inflamed.

◆ Bursitis, inflammation of the bursa, small, fluid-filled sacs that lubricate and cushion pressure points between bones, tendons, and muscles near joints.

◆ Conjunctivitis, inflammation of the conjunctiva, the clear membrane that covers the white part of the eye and lines the inner surface of the eyelids.

◆ Dermatitis, inflammation of the skin. Although there are many different types of dermatitis, it generally describes swollen, reddened, and itchy skin and lesions.

◆ Encephalitis, an inflammation of the brain, usually caused by a virus.

◆ Endocarditis, an infection leading to inflammation of the heart valves and parts of the inside lining of the heart muscle (known as the "endocardium").

◆ Epiglotitis, a life-threatening inflammation of the cartilage that covers the trachea (windpipe).

◆ Hepatitis, inflammation of the liver. Viral hepatitis is inflammation of the liver caused by a virus. There are five identified types of viral hepatitis and each one is caused by a different virus; hepatitis A, hepatitis B, and hepatitis C are the most common types.

◆ Meningitis, inflammation of the membranes (called meninges) surrounding the brain and the spinal cord. People sometimes refer to it as spinal meningitis.

◆ Myocarditis, inflammation or degeneration of the heart muscle.

◆ Myositis is the general term used to describe swelling of the muscles.

◆ Pancreatitis, inflammation of an organ called the pancreas, which makes pancreatic juices and hormones such as insulin. Pancreatic juices contain enzymes that help digest food. Insulin controls the amount of sugar in the blood.

◆ Pericarditis, inflammation of tissue surrounding the heart.

◆ Periodontitis, a disease that involves inflammation of the supporting tissues of the teeth, progressive loss of teeth, and bone loss.

◆ Sclerotitis, inflammation of the membrane that is part of the outer covering of the eyeball.

◆ Sinusitis, inflammation of the sinuses, which are air-filled holes in the bones of the skull.

◆ Temporal arteritis, an inflammatory condition affecting the medium-sized blood vessels that supply the head, eyes, and optic nerves.

◆ Tendonitis, inflammation of the tendons, the tough, flexible bands of tissue that connect your muscles to your bones.

◆ Tonsillitis, an inflammation of the tonsils caused by an infection.

◆ Vasculitis, an inflammation of the blood vessels.

The Least You Need to Know

◆ Inflammation plays a central role in heart disease and strokes.

◆ Most precancerous and cancerous cells show signs of inflammation.

◆ Inflammation is part of or the cause of hundreds of other diseases, including diabetes.

◆ Inflammation may be the switch that turns on Alzheimer's disease.

◆ Inflammation is part of many forms of arthritis and can even affect internal organs.

◆ The damage caused by autoimmune diseases is due to inflammation.

Chapter 3

Fat Is Not Just Fat Anymore

In This Chapter

- ◆ Learn how fat cells cause inflammation
- ◆ How to calculate your BMI
- ◆ How to recognize metabolic syndrome
- ◆ How to measure your waist
- ◆ Recipes for an anti-inflammation diet

Benjamin Franklin said, "I guess I don't so much mind being old, as much as I mind being fat and old." Most of us love to eat, but if we love it too much we get fat. And, like Franklin, we hate getting fat even more than we hate growing older—which we hate a lot.

But fat means more than XXL labels on your clothes. It causes inflammation, puts our lives in jeopardy, and makes us feel physically uncomfortable.

In this chapter, you will learn about the relationship between fat and inflammation, including the discovery that fat actually produces a protein that causes inflammation. You will learn about metabolic syndrome, which can put you at high risk for heart disease and diabetes; how to tell if you are overweight or obese; the surprising risk of malnourishment for people who are overweight; and the benefits of eating whole grains to combat obesity.

New Discoveries About Fat and Inflammation

The fatter you are, the greater the effect on the rest of your body. Up until the last decade we thought of fat as a passive blob of wobbly, unattractive stuff that provided insulation against the cold and greatly affected how we moved and how we looked.

def•i•ni•tion

Hormones act as chemical messengers and are transported to all parts of the body by the bloodstream, where they affect target organs.

An **endocrine organ** is a part of the body that secretes chemicals that control body functions.

However, scientists have learned that fat is much more than that. It actually plays a very important role in our body functions. Fat cells send out chemical signals throughout our bodies, including to our brains, reproductive organs, and immune systems. And researchers are still discovering *hormones* that are made by fat.

Fat is as much a functioning part of your body as your liver or pancreas. In recent years researchers have found that fat is the biggest *endocrine organ* we have, which means that it is the largest part of our bodies that makes hormones.

Scientists have also discovered that human fat cells produce a protein that causes inflammation. This explains why, if you are overweight, you probably have high levels of C-reactive protein (see Chapter 1). Also, we know that being overweight or obese puts your body into an inflammatory state. And too much fat greatly increases the risk of inflammatory diseases such as cancer, diabetes, and arthritis.

Fat: A Modern-Day Disease

As a nation we're getting fat. In the last two decades obesity has risen dramatically in the United States. Nearly two thirds of adults over age 20 are obese or overweight. (It is interesting that the proportion of men who are overweight or obese is higher than the proportion of women in this category.) This fact has prompted some people to suggest that this decade will be known as the obesity decade.

Here are some startling statistics about obesity in the United States.

◆ If we look at obesity alone, one in five (20 percent) of adults 20 years of age and older—over 60 million people—are now obese.

◆ Only a third (33.5 percent) of adults have healthy weights.

◆ The percentage of young people who are overweight has more than tripled since 1980.

Some of the reasons behind the obesity epidemic are:

◆ In general, people drive more and walk less even if they are going short distances.

◆ We use modern appliances rather than our muscles.

◆ We eat ready-made foods and use ready-made ingredients for cooking, which are high in calories, harmful fats, and refined starches, all of which add up to obesity.

◆ Many of our activities are sedentary. We sit and watch TV, use the computer, and play video games rather than walk, run, and play.

◆ Due to advances in technology and machinery, many of our occupations are now sedentary. Jobs involving manual labor are not the norm.

> **Did You Know?**
>
> Among children and teens aged 6 to 19 years, 16 percent are overweight. An additional 15 percent of children and 15 percent of adolescents are at risk of being overweight. And these numbers are quickly rising.

Fat Shortens Life

Many studies show a risk of early death due to obesity. In fact, people who are obese have a 50 to 100 percent increased risk of death from all causes, compared with normal-weight individuals. Most of the high risk is due to heart problems, which, as we know, are closely tied to inflammation.

The National Institutes of Health estimate that the life expectancy of a moderately obese person could be shortened by 2 to 5 years. And over the next few decades, life expectancy for the average American could *decline* by as much as 5 years unless our country's obesity epidemic is stopped.

If you are overweight, losing even 10 to 15 pounds can ease the stress that fat is putting in your body. Experts in obesity recommend about a 10 percent weight loss over 6 months.

Did You Know?

The following are statistics reported by the Surgeon General of the United States:

◆ An estimated 300,000 deaths per year may be attributable to obesity.

◆ The risk of death rises with increasing weight.

◆ Even moderate weight excess (10 to 20 pounds for a person of average height) increases the risk of death, particularly among adults aged 30 to 64 years.

Overweight and Obesity: What Is the Difference?

The standard definition of overweight is an excess of body weight compared to guidelines set by the Centers for Disease Control. The excess weight may come from muscle, bone, fat, and/or body water. Obesity refers specifically to having an abnormally high proportion of body fat.

What the Experts Say

With increasing body mass the risks of heart disease, high blood pressure, gallstones, and Type II diabetes all steadily increase, even among those in the healthy weight category.

—Dr. Walter Willett, author of *Eat, Drink, and Be Healthy*, Free Press, 2001.

To determine whether you are overweight or obese, calculate a number called the body mass index (BMI). This measure is used by most health professionals at this point in time, so it is important to understand it and know how to use it. However, the waist measurement that we describe further on in this chapter is in many ways a better predictor of obesity and the metabolic syndrome, a condition in which a group of risk factors for cardiovascular disease and Type II diabetes occur together. For most people, waist measurement correlates with their amount of body fat.

How to Calculate Your BMI

To determine BMI using pounds and inches, multiply your weight in pounds by 704.5, then divide the result by your height in inches, and divide that result by your height in inches a second time. (Or use the BMI calculator at www.nhlbisupport.com/bmi, or check the following chart.)

An adult who has a BMI between 25 and 29.9 is considered overweight. An adult who has a BMI of 30 or higher is considered obese.

InflamWise

The multiplier 704.5 used for BMI is used by the National Institutes of Health. Other organizations may use a slightly different multiplier. For example, the American Dietetic Association suggests multiplying by 700. The variation in outcome (a few tenths) is insignificant.

For example, by this standard if you are 5 feet 9 inches tall and you weigh between 169 and 202 pounds, your body mass index is 25 to 29.9 and you are considered overweight. If you are 5 feet 9 inches tall and you weigh 203 pounds or more, your body mass is 30 or higher and you are considered obese.

Body Mass Index Table

BMI	Normal						Overweight					Obese										Extreme Obesity														
	19	20	21	22	23	24	25	26	27	28	29	30	31	32	33	34	35	36	37	38	39	40	41	42	43	44	45	46	47	48	49	50	51	52	53	54
Height (inches)												Body Weight (pounds)																								
58	91	96	100	105	110	115	119	124	129	134	138	143	148	153	158	162	167	172	177	181	186	191	196	201	205	210	215	220	224	229	234	239	244	248	253	258
59	94	99	104	109	114	119	124	128	133	138	143	148	153	158	163	168	173	178	183	188	193	198	203	208	212	217	222	227	232	237	242	247	252	257	262	267
60	97	102	107	112	118	123	128	133	138	143	148	153	158	163	168	174	179	184	189	194	199	204	209	215	220	225	230	235	240	245	250	255	261	266	271	276
61	100	106	111	116	122	127	132	137	143	148	153	158	164	169	174	180	185	190	195	201	206	211	217	222	227	232	238	243	248	254	259	264	269	275	280	285
62	104	109	115	120	126	131	136	142	147	153	158	164	169	175	180	186	191	196	202	207	213	218	224	229	235	240	246	251	256	262	267	274	278	284	289	295
63	107	113	118	124	130	135	141	146	152	157	163	169	175	180	186	191	197	203	208	214	220	225	231	237	242	248	254	259	265	270	278	282	287	293	299	304
64	110	116	122	128	134	140	145	151	157	163	169	174	180	186	192	197	204	209	215	221	227	232	238	244	250	256	262	267	273	279	285	282	296	302	308	314
65	114	120	126	132	138	144	150	156	162	168	174	180	186	192	198	204	210	216	222	228	234	240	246	252	258	264	270	276	282	288	294	291	300	312	318	324
66	118	124	130	136	142	148	155	161	167	173	179	186	192	198	204	210	216	223	229	235	241	247	253	260	266	272	278	284	291	297	303	300	315	322	328	334
67	121	127	134	140	146	153	159	166	172	178	185	191	198	204	211	217	223	230	236	242	249	255	261	268	274	280	287	293	299	306	312	319	325	331	338	344
68	125	131	138	144	151	158	164	171	177	184	190	197	203	210	216	223	230	243	243	249	256	262	269	276	282	289	295	302	308	315	322	319	335	341	348	354
69	128	135	142	149	155	162	169	176	182	189	196	203	209	216	223	230	236	250	250	257	263	270	277	284	291	298	304	311	318	324	331	328	345	351	358	365
70	132	139	146	153	160	167	174	181	188	195	202	209	216	222	229	236	243	257	257	264	271	278	285	292	299	306	313	320	327	334	341	348	355	362	369	376
71	136	143	150	157	165	172	179	186	193	200	208	215	222	229	236	243	250	265	265	272	279	286	293	301	308	315	322	329	338	343	351	358	365	372	379	386
72	140	147	154	162	169	177	184	191	199	206	213	221	228	235	242	250	258	272	272	279	287	294	302	309	316	324	331	338	346	353	361	368	375	383	390	397
73	144	151	159	166	174	182	189	197	204	212	219	227	235	242	250	257	265	280	280	288	295	302	310	318	325	333	340	348	355	363	371	378	386	393	401	408
74	148	155	163	171	179	186	194	202	210	218	225	233	241	249	256	264	272	287	287	295	303	311	319	326	334	342	350	358	365	373	381	389	396	404	412	420
75	152	160	168	176	184	192	200	208	216	224	232	240	248	256	264	272	279	287	295	295	303	311	319	327	335	343	351	359	367	375	383	391	399	407	415	423	431
76	156	164	172	180	189	197	205	213	221	230	238	246	254	263	271	279	287	304	304	312	320	328	336	344	353	361	369	377	385	394	402	410	418	426	435	443

Source: Adapted from *Clinical Guidelines on the Identification, Evaluation, and Treatment of Overweight and Obesity in Adults: The Evidence Report.*

To use this BMI table, find your height in the left-hand column labeled "Height." Move across to a given weight. The number at the top of the column is the BMI at that height and weight. Pounds have been rounded off.

InflamWarnings

BMI measurements are not always accurate. If you are muscular you may have a BMI in the overweight range even though you do not have excess body fat. Or if you have low muscle mass you may have a BMI in the healthy weight category—when actually you are undernourished.

BMI, Kids, and Teens

For children and teens, BMI ranges above a normal weight have different labels: at risk of overweight and overweight.

BMI measurement is different for these age groups than for adults. Children's body fat changes over the years as they grow. Also, girls and boys differ in how they store fat as they mature. Therefore BMI for children, also referred to as BMI-for-age, is gender and age specific. BMI-for-age is plotted on gender-specific growth charts. These charts are used for children and teens 2 to 20 years of age. For the 2000 CDC growth charts and additional information, visit the website of the CDC's National Center for Health Statistics, listed in Appendix C.

Overweight and Malnourished

In affluent, developed countries such as the United States, many people have easy access to food and can become overly plump. For the first time in human history, the number of overweight people in the world rivals the number of underweight people, according to a report by the Worldwatch Institute, a Washington, D.C.–based research organization.

And as the world gets fatter we are, ironically, seeing a dramatic increase in malnutrition, which, according to the World Health Organization, is "characterized by obesity and the long-term implications of unbalanced dietary and lifestyle practices that result in chronic diseases such as cardiovascular disease, cancer, and diabetes."

Did You Know?

For every 2-pound increase in weight, the risk of developing arthritis is increased by 9 to 13 percent. In addition, symptoms of arthritis can improve with weight loss.

Source: Arthritis Foundation

The Worldwatch report states that while the world's underfed population has declined recently to 1.1 billion (good news), the number of overweight people has surged to 1.1 billion (bad news). Ironically, people who are overweight, like those who are underweight, often suffer from malnutrition, the definition of which is a lack of nutrients and other important dietary elements needed for maintaining health.

In short, overweight and obese people are often malnourished because they eat a lot of empty calories, such as refined sugar, flour, and grains, which have no nutritional value. Such empty calories abound in fast foods.

According to Gary Gardner, a co-author of the Worldwatch report:

> The hungry and the overweight share high levels of sickness and disability, shortened life expectancies, and lower levels of productivity—each of which is a drag on a country's development. The public health impact is enormous: more than half of the world's disease burden—measured in "years of healthy life lost"—is attributable to hunger, overeating, and widespread vitamin and mineral deficiencies.

If you are a heavy eater of empty-calorie foods, pay attention to the amount of nutrients you eat daily. The author of the highly respected *Eat, Drink, and Be Healthy*, Dr. Walter Willett, suggests taking a multivitamin daily for insurance against vitamin and mineral deficiencies. However, this does not mean that taking multivitamins can give you the freedom to eat junk food. It doesn't work that way. Sound nutrition doesn't come in pills, and multivitamins simply cannot make up for the loss of nutrients found in wholesome foods.

Metabolic Syndrome

One of the major health problems caused by being overweight is metabolic syndrome, a condition that puts people at high risk for Type II diabetes and heart disease. It is also closely linked to inflammation. Fortunately, if the metabolic syndrome is caught early it can be slowed or reversed.

Metabolic syndrome is alarmingly common. One in five (22 percent) U.S. adults has metabolic syndrome, and at least half of persons over age 60 may have the condition, according to the Centers for Disease Control and Prevention. And a recent analysis found that as many as 4.2 percent of teenagers in the United States (aged 12 to 19 years) have the disorder.

What Is Metabolic Syndrome?

Metabolic syndrome is a collection of problems that put people at high risk for serious disease. It is closely linked to obesity. The exact cause of the syndrome is not known, but it is believed to be a disorder of metabolism, the complicated process of breaking down and converting the liquids we drink and the foods we eat into substances that the body needs to function.

If you carry fat mainly around your waist, you are more likely to develop metabolic syndrome than if you carry it in your hips and thighs. You have probably heard these weight distributions described as apple shapes versus pear shapes.

Key features of metabolic syndrome are:

◆ Fat around the stomach. Scientists call this central adiposity; the rest of us know it as a pot belly.

◆ High blood pressure.

◆ High blood fats (triglycerides).

◆ Difficulty in processing your body's sugar.

◆ Low numbers of the good cholesterol, HDL.

If you have three or more of these conditions, you probably, or most likely, have metabolic syndrome and are high risk for heart disease.

Metabolic Syndrome and Inflammation

Chronic inflammation goes hand and hand with metabolic syndrome. The present scientific knowledge about the connection between the two is that stomach fat actually makes chemical substances called cytokines which cause the liver to make CRP (see Chapter 1). Also, the more features of the metabolic syndrome you have, the higher your CRP level.

What Causes Metabolic Syndrome?

The easy answer to what sets off metabolic syndrome is: genetic makeup, what you eat, and your exercise habits. In other words, if you have a family tendency to put on fat around your waist and you don't control the problem, you are a strong candidate for metabolic syndrome.

How to Measure Your Waist

A waist measurement determines metabolic syndrome even if other measurements such as body mass index fall within the normal range. To measure your waist, place a tape measure around your bare abdomen just above your hip bone. Be sure that the tape is snug, but not too snug. Do not pull it tight. You should not feel pressure on your skin. Also, the tape should be parallel to the floor. (It should not follow your belt line, and thus is not the same as your belt size.) Relax and breathe out. Do not breathe in. That is cheating! Measure your waist.

Women with a waist measurement of more than 35 inches or men with a waist measurement of more than 40 inches are high risk for metabolic syndrome.

Tackling Metabolic Syndrome

The American Heart Association recommends lifestyle therapies as the first-line interventions to reduce the risk of developing metabolic syndrome. These lifestyle interventions include:

- Weight loss to achieve a desirable weight

- Increased physical activity, with a goal of at least 30 minutes of moderate-intensity activity on most days of the week

- Healthy eating habits that include reduced intake of saturated fat, trans fats, and cholesterol

Dr. S. Sethu Reddy, an endocrinologist at the Cleveland Clinic Foundation, says that "the best medication for metabolic syndrome is common sense." For instance, studies have shown that small decreases in weight—even in persons who are obese—can result in significant improvements in markers of metabolic syndrome. "It all comes down to lifestyle choices," says Dr. Reddy.

Sound familiar? In other words, follow the anti-inflammation diet and lifestyle. The diet is discussed later in this chapter, as well as in Chapter 4.

Metabolic Syndrome and Your Brain

Research shows that people with metabolic syndrome and high levels of inflammation are very high risk for the brain-robbing condition dementia. A recent study led by Dr. Kristine Yaffe of the University of California at San Francisco of more than 2,600 men and women in their 70s found that after 5 years, those with metabolic syndrome were 20 percent more likely to develop signs of cognitive impairment, including memory loss, than those without metabolic syndrome. Those with both metabolic syndrome *and* high levels of inflammation were 66 percent more likely to suffer from mental impairment.

Did You Know?
If you're over 50, you have a better than one in three chance of having metabolic syndrome. The rate of people with metabolic syndrome has soared by more than 60 percent in the last decade, paralleling the steep rise in obesity among Americans young and old.

Eat an Anti-Inflammation Diet to Prevent Metabolic Syndrome

The best protection against metabolic syndrome is to lose weight and eat a health-promoting diet. Studies show that eating a Mediterranean-style diet, such as the anti-inflammation approach, and maintaining a healthful weight can keep metabolic syndrome away. That means foods that come from plants: grains, vegetables, fruits, beans, legumes, nuts, and olive oil. Added advantages of these foods are their high nutritional value, so that if you are overweight you will not also be malnourished.

Follow the Anti-Inflammation Diet if You Have Metabolic Syndrome

If you already have metabolic syndrome, the best thing you can do is get your weight down.

Eat Whole Grains to Prevent Metabolic Syndrome

Scientists at Tufts University found that following a diet rich in whole-grain foods can delay development of the metabolic syndrome. Earlier studies found that eating whole grains reduced the risk of developing metabolic syndrome among middle-aged people. The scientists also found that people who consumed high amounts of refined grains had twice the risk of having metabolic syndrome than those people who consumed only small amounts.

Whole grains are not only good for you, they are delicious. We give more details about them in Chapter 8. In the meantime, here are some delicious recipes to whet your appetite.

Big Protein Red Quinoa Salad

Makes about 4 cups

Quinoa is a grain that comes from the Andes Mountains of South America. Quinoa contains more protein than any other grain.

¾ cup red quinoa	1 TB. chopped fresh dill
1½ cups water	½ cup chopped fresh parsley
1 tsp. minced garlic	½ cup organic golden raisins
2 TB. extra-virgin olive oil	½ cup organic hazelnuts, lightly toasted and coarsely chopped
¼ cup fresh lemon juice	
2 tsp. minced or grated lemon zest	¼ cup thinly sliced green onions
½ cup peeled, seeded, and ¼-inch-diced organic cucumber	¼ cup grated carrot
	¾–1 tsp. sea salt
½ cup canned organic garbanzo beans, drained	¼ tsp. black pepper

Rinse quinoa in cold water and drain well. Put the drained quinoa in a heavy medium saucepan and dry roast the grain over medium heat, stirring occasionally for about 1 minute. Add the water, bring to a boil, then reduce to a simmer and cover with a tight-fitting lid. Cook for about 15 minutes or until all water is absorbed.

Remove from the heat and let stand, covered, for 10 minutes. Remove lid, fluff grains with a fork, and let cool to room temperature.

In a large bowl, combine the cooked quinoa with the remaining ingredients and toss well.

Reprinted with permission from Kathy Casey Food Studios.

Wild Rice Azteca

Makes 6–8 side-dish servings

Wild rice is highly nutritious. It is not actually rice, but an annual water-grass seed, naturally abundant in the cold rivers and lakes of Minnesota and Canada. Wild rice was a staple in the diet of the Chippewa and Sioux Indians.

3½ cup reduced-sodium chicken broth	1 (14.5-oz.) can diced tomatoes, drained
¾ cup wild rice	1 canned chipotle chili, minced*
¾ cup jasmine or other long-grain rice	1 tsp. ground cumin
2 TB. olive oil	⅓ cup minced fresh cilantro
1 medium onion, chopped	Optional: Avocado
2 cloves garlic, minced or pressed	

In a 4- to 5-quart saucepan, bring broth to a boil over high heat. Add wild rice; reduce heat to low, cover tightly and simmer until grains begin to open and feel tender to bite, about 45 minutes.

Stir in jasmine rice. Cover tightly, and simmer until jasmine and wild rice are tender to bite and liquid is absorbed, 20 to 25 more minutes.

While wild and jasmine rices cook, heat olive oil in a 10- to 12-inch skillet over medium-high heat. Add onion, garlic, diced tomatoes, chipotle, and cumin to oil. Reduce heat to medium and stir until heated through, about 5 minutes.

When rice is done, remove from heat and gently stir in onion-tomato mixture and minced cilantro until blended. Garnish each serving with avocado slices (optional).

*A second chipotle chili can be added to increase spiciness.

Courtesy of Oldways and the Whole Grains Council, www. wholegrainscouncil.org.

Bulgur and Black Bean Salad

Makes 4 servings

Bulgur is a quick-cooking form of whole wheat that has been cleaned, parboiled, dried, ground into particles, and sifted into distinct sizes. It is versatile and has a pleasant, nutlike flavor.

1 cup uncooked bulgur	**6 stalks green onions, chopped in small pieces (green and white parts)**
1 orange (or lemon)	
1 (14–15-oz.) can black beans, drained and rinsed thoroughly	**4 TB. fresh parsley, chopped**
	2 tsp. vinegar
1 red bell pepper, chopped in small pieces	**2 TB. canola or olive oil**
	½ tsp. ground cumin

Put 1 cup bulgur and 2 cups water in covered saucepan. Bring to boil then simmer 12-15 minutes until excess liquid is absorbed.

Scrub orange, then grate the rind off. Cut orange in half and squeeze juice into a large mixing bowl. Add orange rind, vinegar, oil and cumin to the orange juice in the bowl. Chop all the vegetables while the bulgur is cooking.

Throw vegetables and rinsed beans in the bowl and mix. Add cooked bulgur and mix again.

Add any vegetables you want. Also try using a lemon instead of an orange.

Courtesy of Oldways and the Whole Grains Council, www. wholegrainscouncil.org.

Mushroom Brown Rice Pilaf

Makes 4 generous servings or 6 smaller servings

Brown rice has its bran, germ, and endosperm intact, and is chewier and slower-cooking than milled white rice. It is nutritious and has fewer calories per ounce in this nutty rice, as well. The brown grains come in long and short, which are interchangeable. Some cooks like to toast if first to achieve a nuttier flavor.

½ large onion, chopped	**1 cup brown rice**
1 cup sliced mushrooms (4–5 mushrooms)	**2 cups chicken or vegetable broth**
1 TB. olive or canola oil	

Heat the oil in a large saucepan and brown onion and mushrooms for about 5 minutes. Add brown rice and stir to coat grains in oil. Add broth, bring to a boil, and then turn down to a simmer.

Simmer for about 45 minutes or until all liquid is absorbed. Cooking time for whole-grain rice varies according to the variety of rice; check package directions.

You can make a pilaf like this with any grain—not just rice.

Simply vary the amount of broth and the cooking time according to the different grain.

In a hurry? Try bulgur or quinoa; both cook in less than 15 minutes.

Courtesy of Oldways and the Whole Grains Council, www. wholegrainscouncil.org.

Spinach Pasta Salad

Makes 4 servings

Whole-grain pasta comes in a lot of varieties. You might want to try rice or corn pasta in this recipe as well.

6 oz. uncooked whole-wheat, whole-rice, or quinoa/corn pasta

2 TB. lemon juice (or juice of half a lemon)

3 TB. olive oil

2 tsp. minced garlic (2 cloves)

4 cups fresh spinach leaves, cleaned and chopped

1 15-oz. can chickpeas or other white beans, drained and rinsed

2 oz. feta cheese

Bring a large saucepan of water to a boil, and cook pasta according to package directions. (Spiral whole-wheat pasta is good, and takes about 8 minutes to cook.)

In a large salad bowl, mix the lemon juice, oil, and garlic. (Minced garlic in a jar is handy!) While the pasta boils, clean and chop spinach, and drain and rinse beans. Drain pasta and mix with dressing in the salad bowl. Add spinach, beans, and feta and mix.

Chill for 1 hour or more, or simply enjoy it warm, with salt and pepper to taste.

Courtesy of Oldways and the Whole Grains Council, www. wholegrainscouncil.org.

Curried Barley and Raisins

Makes 4 servings

Barley's not just for soups! You can add shrimp, chicken, or other lean protein to this recipe and make it into a one-dish meal.

½ cup lightly pearled barley	1 tsp. curry powder
2 cups broth or water	2 TB. raisins
2 tsp. olive oil	2 TB. fresh parsley, chopped
1 large onion (about 2 cups), in thin slices	(The above three amounts are approximate. You decide!)
1 tsp. minced garlic	2 TB. slivered almonds, toasted

Cook the barley in the broth or water for about 45 minutes, until liquid is absorbed.

While the barley cooks, sauté the onion in the oil in a very large skillet for about 15 minutes, until golden brown, stirring occasionally.

Add garlic and curry powder, mix, and cook 1 more minute to blend spices.

When barley is done, add it to the skillet and mix thoroughly so barley gets coated with delicious spices and oil.

Turn off heat and add raisins, parsley, and almonds. Add salt and pepper to taste.

Courtesy of Oldways and the Whole Grains Council, www. wholegrainscouncil.org.

Armenian Christmas Pudding

Makes 4 servings

Bulgur is a dried, parcooked wheat popular in the Near East. It's mild in flavor and quick-cooking, making it perfect as a side dish—or even, as here, as an ingredients for a traditional Armenian holiday dish.

1 quart water	**½ cup apricots, diced**
½ cup bulgur (coarse bulgur is best, but any bulgur will do)	**½ cup dates, diced**
	¼ cup sugar
½ cup raisins	

Cook bulgur, raisins, apricots, and dates in water for 20 minutes. Add sugar and cook an additional 15 minutes. Pour into bowl or individual serving bowls.

Garnish with walnuts, blanched almonds, and a small pinch of cinnamon.

Courtesy of Oldways and the Whole Grains Council, www. wholegrainscouncil.org. Recipe by Sunnyland Mills

No Butter! Apple Cranberry Pie

Makes 6 servings

This pie has no crust, so it's quick and healthy. Mix it by hand with a large spoon, so the apples don't get crushed.

1 egg

½ cup sugar

½ cup whole-wheat flour (regular or pastry)

1 tsp. baking powder

¼ tsp. salt

½ tsp. cinnamon

¼ tsp. vanilla

3 small or 2 large apples, cored and chopped but not peeled

½ cup dried cranberries

1 cup chopped nuts (walnuts or pecans are good)

Preheat oven to 350°F. Spray a 10-inch pie pan with cooking spray. In a large bowl, beat egg thoroughly with a fork, until it forms a ribbon. Add sugar, flour, baking powder, salt, cinnamon, and vanilla, and mix thoroughly with a large spoon. Add apples, cranberries, and nuts, and mix as well as you can with a large spoon. You'll wonder if you've done something wrong, as it's a very lumpy mix—not even qualifying for the word "batter." But soldier on, and mix as best you can. After 4 to 5 minutes of elbow grease, suddenly it all hangs together.

Toss it all in the pie plate and bake at 350°F for 30 minutes.

Serve warm or cool.

Courtesy of Oldways and the Whole Grains Council, www. wholegrainscouncil.org. Recipe by Cynthia Harriman.

The Least You Need to Know

◆ Fat cells cause inflammation.

◆ You can be overweight and malnourished at the same time.

◆ If you have a fat waist you may have metabolic syndrome.

◆ Your waist measurement determines whether you have metabolic syndrome— even if your BMI is normal.

◆ Eating whole-grain foods frequently can delay metabolic syndrome.

Part 2

Diet and Inflammation

In this part, we explain the seven principles of the anti-inflammation diet and how they work. Following basic information about the diet, separate chapters cover each of the principles and explain how they work to reduce inflammation. The chapters also give you practical tips on how to make the principles work. We even include a chapter on how nutritional needs change as we grow up and grow older. If you follow these principles, you will reduce the risk of not just one, but many life-threatening and debilitating diseases.

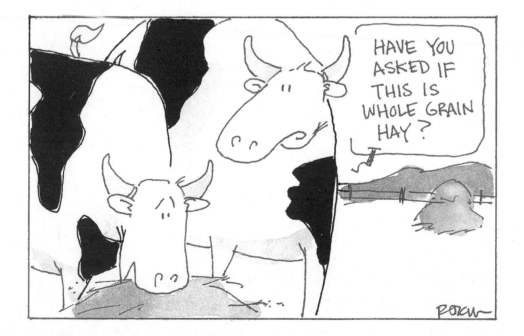

4

The Seven Principles of the Anti-Inflammation Diet

In This Chapter

- ◆ The seven principles explained
- ◆ Why you should eliminate trans fats from your diet
- ◆ The importance of omega-3 fatty acids in your diet

The anti-inflammation diet is based on scientific studies and common sense. When you follow this path to health, you are eating a balance of wholesome foods and calories rich in nutrients.

As we mentioned in Chapter 1, the point of the anti-inflammation diet is to eat foods that taste great and are great for you. The diet has seven major principles:

1. Eat a well-balanced variety of wholesome foods.

2. Keep away from saturated and trans fats.

3. Eat one good source of omega-3 fatty acids every day.

4. Eat a lot of whole grains.

5. Eat lean sources of protein.

6. Eat plenty of fruits and vegetables.

7. Eliminate processed and refined foods as much as possible.

Starting with eating a balanced diet, this chapter covers the facts behind the seven principles.

Principle #1—Eat a Well-Balanced Variety of Wholesome Foods

Balance is your key to a healthful diet. Eating a variety of foods means that you will not lack in the nutrients your body requires to stay healthy and function well.

Balanced diets include *macronutrients*, which include carbohydrates, protein, and fat, as well as vitamins, minerals, and fiber in the correct proportions. Here are just a few examples of what can happen when diets are out of balance:

def•i•ni•tion

Macronutrients are those nutrients required in large amounts for normal growth and development.

Food has three types of macronutrients: carbohydrates, protein, and fat. Each one provides important benefits but can also present problems for your body if you eat the wrong kind or you consume too much of any one given type.

◆ People who do not take in enough calories lack energy and feel fatigued. If they take in too many calories they get fat (and will also lack energy and feel fatigued).

◆ Children who do not eat enough protein do not grow as they should. Adults who do not get enough protein do not heal well after injuries.

◆ People who eat too many of the wrong kinds of fats develop inflammation and are at high risk for heart disease. People who eat too little of the good fats are also high risk for heart disease.

Helpful tips for a balanced diet that follows the healthy eating guidelines are presented in Chapter 5.

Principle #2—Eat Only Unsaturated Fats

One of the major things you can do to control inflammation is to watch what types of fat you eat and drink. This does not mean following a low-fat diet, which has been shown to have marginal health benefits. It means paying attention to what type and how much fat you eat.

In order to understand how important fats are to your health, it is helpful to know some basic things about them.

Fats 101

Fats are tasty—they are one of the key ingredients that make foods enjoyable. They also give us the feeling of fullness that keeps hunger pangs away. Because of the satisfaction they deliver, most of us tend to get plenty of fat in our diets.

The building blocks of fats are "essential" fatty acids. Our bodies cannot make them; they must be obtained from food. Fatty acids supply our bodies with the raw materials that help control inflammation, blood pressure, blood clotting, and other key body functions.

The following table lists key details about the fats that you should pay attention to in your diet.

Bad Fats

- Saturated fats: These are the nutritional culprits behind high LDL levels (bad cholesterol). Saturated fats are found in animal products such as butter, cheese, whole milk, ice cream, cream, and fatty meats. They are also found in coconut, palm, and palm kernel oils. They have a flavor that most of us love.

- Trans fatty acids: These fats result from turning liquid vegetable oil into a solid, a procedure called hydrogenation. In the process, the fats are changed from being mainly unsaturated to being mainly saturated. Trans fats raise LDL levels (bad cholesterol) and lower HDL levels (good cholesterol). They are found in a long list of foods, including fried foods, commercially baked goods (donuts, cookies, and crackers), processed foods, and margarines.

Good Fats

- Unsaturated fats: These fats help to lower blood cholesterol if used in place of saturated fats. There are two types: monounsaturated and polyunsaturated (see below).

- Monounsaturated fats: These fats help to lower blood cholesterol if used in place of saturated fats. Olive oil is the most popular monounsaturated fat.

- Polyunsaturated fats: These fats can be found in safflower, sunflower, corn, and soybean oils.

The Devil Is in the Details

Whether a fat is beneficial or harmful depends on its type, not how much you eat. This fact was confirmed by researchers at Harvard University, who found no link between the percentage of daily calories consumed from fat and any disease including cancer, heart disease, and obesity.

But the devil is in the details. When fats carry the label "saturated," they can lead to heart disease and other problems. And trans fats are the worst.

A case in point: an analysis by Harvard University researchers found that replacing only 30 calories (7 grams) of carbohydrates every day with 30 calories (4 grams) of trans fats nearly *doubled* the risk for heart disease. Plain old saturated fats increased risk as well, but not nearly as much.

In contrast, eating either monounsaturated or polyunsaturated fats has the opposite effect. The researchers found that replacing 80 calories of carbohydrates with 80 calories of either of these good fats every day lowers the risk for heart disease by 30 or 40 percent.

The following sections cover some of the facts about fats that you should know to maximize the effectiveness of the anti-inflammatory diet.

Saturated Fats

Saturated fats are harmful fats. They greatly increase the risk of cardiovascular disease. Saturated fats are usually solid or almost solid at room temperature. All animal fats, such as those in meat, poultry, and dairy products, are saturated. Processed and fast foods are also saturated. Palm, palm kernel, and coconut oils are naturally saturated.

The American Heart Association recommends that you limit your saturated fat intake to 7 to 10 percent of total calories (or less) each day. We'd like it to be even lower than that.

The Worst of the Lot: Trans Fats

Trans fats are created when liquid oils are made into solids. These fats abound in processed foods because they add to their shelf life and increase flavor.

Girl Scout cookies, french fries, and even Saltines are high in trans fats. They make up a whopping 40 percent of the ingredients in snack crackers. They are found in enormous amounts in fast foods such as fried chicken, biscuits, fried fish sandwiches, pies, donuts, and muffins, and in packaged processed foods such as crackers, most cookies, cake, cake icing, toaster pastries, microwave popcorn, canned biscuits, and instant latte coffee drinks.

According to scientific findings by the Institute of Medicine, "It is recommended that trans fatty acid consumption be as low as possible while consuming a nutritionally adequate diet." In addition, Dr. Jeffrey Aron of the University of California at San Francisco puts his advice on trans fats this way: "There should be a warning label on food made with this stuff like there is with nicotine. It's that bad for you."

Did You Know?

Replacing partially hydrogenated fat in the U.S. diet with natural unhydrogenated veg-etable oils would prevent approximately 30,000 premature coronary deaths per year, according to the Harvard School of Public Health. Other evidence suggests this number is closer to 100,000 premature deaths annually.

New research from Harvard's Nurses' Health Study shows that trans fatty acids are linked to an increase in inflammation throughout the body, especially in women who are overweight. Even small amounts can significantly increase the rate of heart attacks.

The Harvard study also found that women who ate the most trans fatty acids had a 53 percent increased risk of coronary heart disease compared to those who ate the least. A recent 10-year study showed similar results. Men who ate the most trans fats had twice the risk of heart attack.

It is startling that these large increases in risk occur with as little as a 2 to 3 percent increase in calories or 4 to 6 grams of trans fatty acids daily.

As of January 1, 2006, the amount of trans fats in a food must be listed on product labels. And healthier products such as trans-fat-free microwave popcorn are becoming more available.

 InflamWarnings _____

According to the Food and Drug Administration, a product claiming to have zero trans fat can actually contain up to a half gram. (Canada set a different standard of zero as under 0.2 grams.) That means if you eat two servings, which is easy to do, you are actually taking in a gram of trans fat. So when food shopping be sure to check the ingredient lists of all foods you are considering. Look for partially hydrogenated vegetable oil and vegetable shortening even if the product claims to have no trans fats. If they are listed, search for another product that does not have these bad fats.

Monounsaturated Fats

Monounsaturated fats are known as good fats because they lower levels of bad cholesterol and raise levels of good cholesterol. They can benefit your health greatly when you use them in place of saturated fats.

Monounsaturated fats are liquid at room temperature, but may solidify in the refrigerator. Foods high in monounsaturated fat include olive, peanut, and canola oils.

The Polys

You could not live without polyunsaturated fatty acids (PUFA). They are what nutritionists call "essential nutrients" for the human body. However, it is a quirk of human physiology that our bodies cannot produce them—we have to get them from what we eat and drink.

We require two types of PUFAs to live—omega-3s and omega-6s. They each play their own important roles, and the balance between them is very important. In general terms, they both make hormones that lead to and control inflammation. Omega-6's hormones create inflammation; omega-3's hormones quiet inflammation.

Unfortunately, it is much harder to find and consume the omega-3s than the omega-6s:

- Omega-6s are found in oils from certain seeds and the fat of animals fed on grains.
- Omega-3s are in oily fish from cold waters, leafy greens, certain seeds and nuts, flax, hemp, certain vegetable oils, and sea vegetables.

For more information about omega-3 and omega-6 fatty acids, see Principle #3.

The following table lists the proportion of different fats in commonly eaten foods. Note how easy it is to consume a lot of trans fatty acids. For example, on any given day if you had a couple of pieces of toast with a tablespoon of margarine for breakfast, a sandwich with fries for lunch, and four chocolate-cream cookies for an afternoon snack, you'd be at 8 grams of trans fats before you even reached for the cheese and crackers to accompany your evening cocktail.

In comparison, using olive, canola, or safflower oil throughout the day to prepare foods and in salad dressings keeps your diet on a healthful path.

Oils	Amount	Saturated	Monounsaturated	Polyunsaturated	Trans
Canola	1 TB.	1 g	8 g	4 g	0
Canola for frying (partially hydrogenated)	1 TB.	1 g	10 g	2 g	4 g
French fries (McDonald's)	1 medium serving	3 g	8 g	5 g	4 g
Margarine (spread)	1 oz.	3 g	5 g	6 g	1 g
Margarine (hard)	1 TB.	2 g	5 g	3 g	3 g
Olive oil	1 TB.	2 g	10 g	1 g	0 g
Chocolate-cream cookies	1	–	1 g	–	1 g
Safflower	1 TB.	1 g	10 g	2 g	0 g
Saltines (crushed)	1 cup	1 g	5 g	1 g	3 g

Source: NutritionData.com; USDA National Nutrient Database for Standard Reference, Release 18.

Principle #3—Eat One Good Source of Omega-3 Fatty Acids Every Day

Several decades ago, researchers studied the Eskimos living in the Artic, who rarely developed heart disease or rheumatoid arthritis. Curiously, the scientists discovered that the amount of total fat in the Eskimo diet is similar to that of a Western-style diet.

Pursuing the mystery further, researchers found the catch: the *source* of fat is different in the Artic diet versus the Western diet. The fat that Eskimos eat comes primarily from marine mammals and fish. Westerners get their fat from land animals and plants.

These early studies led to more research to find which nutrient in fish oils was boosting the health of the Eskimos. The answer? Omega-3 fatty acids. Since the early studies of Eskimos, many other investigations have confirmed that omega-3 fatty acids have a positive effect on health.

Omega-3s not only decrease inflammation, but they also prevent irregular heartbeats, reduce plaque in artery walls, and decrease blood clotting, blood fats, and blood pressure. And inflammatory diseases such as rheumatoid arthritis, ulcerative colitis, and Crohn's disease appear to improve with omega-3s.

It seems like the powers of omega-3s are endless. Studies have also found or suggested that they do the following:

◆ Reduce the risk of diabetes.

◆ Reduce insulin resistance in people with diabetes.

◆ Increase bone density.

◆ Lower the risk of breast, prostate, and colon cancer.

◆ Improve the skin in people with a condition called psoriasis.

◆ Improve cognition and visual acuity.

◆ In children, boost levels of the brain chemicals serotonin and dopamine.

Researchers at the National Academy of Sciences, which usually sets the government's standards for nutrition, are so enthusiastic about omega-3 fatty acids that they have established a minimum daily requirement for them: 1.1 grams for adult women and 1.6 grams for adult men.

And the American Heart Association urges everyone to eat at least two small (3-ounce) servings of fish a week. It is particularly important after menopause in women and after age 45 in men, when coronary risk increases.

InflamWise

If you are concerned about mercury and other contaminants in seafood, you might consider getting your omega-3s from plant oils such as flax, walnuts, or canola oil.

The American Heart Association also advises people who already have heart disease to consume about 1 gram a day of omega-3 fatty acids. To manage this amount, most people have to take a supplement. This is a rare departure from protocol for a major health organization—they rarely endorse dietary supplements.

There are three important omega-3 fatty acids. EPA and DHA are found in large quantities in fish oils. Plant oils also contain another fatty acid called ALA, which your body must convert to DHA and EPA.

The three omega-3 fatty acids—EPA, DHA, and ALA—are alike in some ways and different in others. ALA is derived from plant oils. EPA and DHA are derived from marine mammals. All three block a compound that causes inflammation. They also keep the body's cell membranes flexible and elastic.

The omega-3 fat is particularly important. Infants need DHA to develop properly. Aging adults need DHA to stay sharp mentally. A study of 815 seniors living in Chicago found that those with the highest levels of DHA were the least likely to have Alzheimer's disease. ALA was also protective, but not EPA.

DHA and EPA are found mainly in fatty fish like herring, salmon, mackerel, and blue-fin tuna, and the fish oil supplements made from them.

ALA is found mainly in flax seeds and walnuts and in plant oils like flax, canola, and soybean. Flax seeds and flax oil are the richest sources of ALA. Flax-enriched eggs, along with some fish like Atlantic salmon and canned sardines, are good sources of ALA. Small amounts of ALA are found in products made with added flax like cereals, breads, bagels, spaghetti, energy bars, and cookies. Beef, pork, and chicken also contain small amounts of ALA because livestock and poultry ingest ALA in their daily rations.

The table below lists foods that the U.S. Department of Agriculture allows to claim as high in, or excellent sources of, the three types of omega-3 fats.

ALA	EPA
Flax oil	Herring
Flaxseeds	Salmon, coho, wild
Walnuts	Mackerel
Walnut oil	Salmon, Atlantic/wild
Canola oil	Tuna, bluefin
Soybean oil	Sardines, canned/oil
Omega-3 enriched eggs	Menhaden oil capsules
Atlantic salmon	Shark
Sardines, canned in oil	Striped bass/sea bass

DHA

Salmon, Atlantic/wild	Sea bass
Tuna, bluefin	Shark
Herring	Sardines, canned/oil
Salmon, coho/wild	Menhaden oil capsules
Striped bass	Omega-3 enriched eggs
Mackerel	

Source: Flax Council of Canada

The 3/6 Balancing Act

Like omega-3s, omega-6 fatty acids are essential. They are necessary for life, but our bodies do not produce them naturally, so we have to get them from the foods we eat. Although omega-6 fatty acids are necessary for us, they also promote inflammation and blood clotting, and they have been connected to a long list of diseases including prostate cancer, heart disease, and diabetes.

One of the components of omega-6 fatty acids is arachidonic acid (AA), which plays a key role in inflammatory conditions. Our bodies change AA into inflammation-producing hormones. Under normal circumstances AA is a friend that we rely on to protect and heal us. However, when AA is out of balance it can lead to inflammation that spirals out of control.

Because of our love of processed and fast foods over the past 50 years, most Americans get way too much omega-6 fatty acid in their diets, which essentially blocks the absorption of omega-3 fatty acids. Omega-6 fatty acids are found in safflower, soybean, and corn oils, which are in many processed foods. Omega-6s have largely replaced omega-3s in the modern diet.

Scientists do not agree about the ideal ratio of omega-6 to omega-3 fatty acids that we should consume. And some nutritionists say that a specific ratio is not what matters, but that it is important to greatly increase the amount of omega-3s we eat.

InflamWise

Lower your intake of AA to lower your blood pressure. According to a new study of 4,680 people age 40 to 59, the lower your consumption of foods high in AA, the lower your blood pressure.

However, Dr. Walter Willett, one of the most prominent nutritionists in the country, if not the most prominent, says, "Given the wide-ranging importance and benefits of omega-3 fatty acids, try to eat at least one good source of them a day."

Principle #4—Eat a Lot of Whole Grains

It might have been the puffy white stuff or delicate slices made for tea sandwiches, but it is a good bet that you grew up eating white bread. You also probably ate refined rice and turned your nose up at the nutritious brown stuff. We all did. Sadly, the American tradition of eating refined foods has worked against us nutritionally. While supplying a large part of our daily food intake, refined foods have little nutritional value and many empty calories.

Ironically, the word refined means "free from impurities," when, actually, refining grains ends up making them "free of nutrition." All of the good-for-you stuff is refined out of the food.

When you hear the words "whole grains" suggested as an alternative to refined grains, you may think "BLAH! I might as well eat sticks and rocks." The truth is whole grains can be delicious. And they pack a powerful nutritional punch.

Whole grains have disease-fighting phytochemicals and antioxidants, which are thought to provide protection against disease, as well as B vitamins, vitamin E, magnesium, iron, and fiber. People who eat whole grains regularly have lower cholesterol levels and less risk of heart disease. And, as we discussed in the previous chapter, they can prevent obesity.

Whole grains are so powerful that the U.S. Food and Drug Administration recommends that people eat more of them, and has created rules on what foods distributors can label as whole grain. Eating whole grains has also gotten support from a number of other major health organizations. The American Heart Association, the U.S. Department of Health and Human Services, and the Healthy People 2010 Report all recommend three or more servings of whole grains per day.

> **Did You Know?**
>
> People who eat three daily servings of whole grains have been shown to have a lower risk of heart disease by 25 to 36 percent, stroke by 37 percent, Type II diabetes by 21 to 27 percent, digestive system cancers by 21 to 43 percent, and hormone-related cancers by 10 to 40 percent.

What Is a Whole Grain?

Whole grains are the intact seed of a plant. The seed is made up of three key parts: the bran, the germ, and the endosperm. When grains are refined, parts of the seeds are removed. Whole grains include wheat, corn, rice, oats, barley, quinoa, and others when they are eaten in their "whole" form.

InflamWarnings

Just because a package says "whole grain" does not mean that it is. Be careful: food producers sometimes print "whole grain" on products that contain only very small amounts of them. To avoid being fooled by this false advertising, be sure to look closely at the ingredients lists on product packages. If the first ingredient listed does not say "whole," it is not a good source.

Principle #5—Eat Healthy Sources of Protein

Protein is the middle child of nutritional research—it receives little attention in comparison to fats and carbohydrates. However, protein is necessary for physical development, health, and life itself. And it is an important source of energy.

The Institute of Medicine recommends a daily allowance for protein of 7 grams a day per 20 pounds of body weight. For a 130-pound woman that means 45.5 grams a day, roughly equivalent to a 1.5-ounce bag of walnuts.

Some of the protein we eat contains all the essential amino acids, which are to protein what fatty acids are to fat. They are the building blocks of protein that humans need to live but cannot make on their own. Complete proteins contain all of the amino acids we need. As a general rule, animal proteins are complete.

Other sources of protein come from fruits, vegetables, grains, and nuts. They are called incomplete proteins because, with one exception, they lack at least one of the essential amino acids. This is an important fact for vegetarians who must get the essential amino acids from a balance of protein-containing foods.

Animal products differ greatly in the amount of fat they contain. For example, a 3-ounce lean hamburger has 22 grams of protein and 13 grams of fat, 5 of which are saturated fat. In contrast, 3 ounces of cooked chicken with no skin has 25 grams of protein, 3 grams of fat, and less than a gram of saturated fat.

There are also large differences in the amount of fat in animal versus plant sources of protein. Three ounces of cooked black beans have 9 grams of protein and no fat.

If you love meat, pick only the leanest cuts. Fish, poultry, beans, nuts, and many whole grains are less fatty choices of protein. For more information on this topic, see Chapter 9.

Principle #6—Eat Plenty of Fruits and Vegetables

Fruits and vegetables are the foundation of a healthy diet. Research has proven that they are critical to good health. For example, scientists at Harvard University followed the health and dietary habits of 110,000 participants for 14 years. Those who ate eight or more servings of fruits and vegetables a day were 30 percent less likely to have a heart attack or stroke.

What the Experts Say

One reason why having more fruits and vegetables is good is that if you eat them, you are likely to eat less beef and other high-fat foods such as other meats and desserts. Plus, the fiber in fruits and vegetables bind to cholesterol and help remove it from the blood.

—Dr. Richard L. Harvey, medical director of the Rehabilitation Institute of Chicago.

Fruits and vegetables are perfect fast foods. Instead of reaching for chips, have carrot sticks. Instead of a candy bar, grab an apple. You get the picture.

According to Dr. Walter Willet, who led the study mentioned above, although all fruits and vegetables are likely to contribute to heart and stroke prevention, the following are particularly important: green leafy vegetables, such as lettuce, spinach, Swiss chard, and mustard greens; cruciferous vegetables, such as broccoli, cauliflower, cabbage, Brussels sprouts, bok choy, and kale; and citrus fruits, such as oranges, lemons, limes, and grapefruit (and their juices) make important contributions.

Did You Know?

Increasing fruit and vegetable intake by as little as one serving per day can have a real impact on heart disease risk. Studies by Harvard University found that for every extra serving of fruits and vegetables that participants added to their diets, their risk of heart disease dropped by 4 percent.

In this principle we recommend that you eat plenty of fruits and vegetables. How many is plenty? Most people need to double the amount of fruits and vegetables they eat every day. The national five-to-nine-a-day program recommends that little kids (ages 2 to 6) eat a minimum of five servings a day. Older kids, teenage girls, and active women should eat at least seven. Teenage boys and active men should eat at least nine servings a day.

Principle #7—Eliminate Refined and Processed Foods as Much as Possible

Refined flour, rice, and sugar are all empty calories (see Chapter 3) that lead to obesity, diabetes, and other severe health problems. Need we say more? Eliminate them from your diet whenever possible.

Refined foods are omnipresent in processed foods. Food processing strips foods of their nutrients. Often fat, sugar, sodium, additives, and preservatives are added in. Examples of processed or refined foods are: frozen meals, prepackaged meals, fried foods, cakes, cookies, canned biscuits, chips, breakfast bars, toaster treats, white flour, white bread, white rice, white pasta, sodas, juice with sugar, margarine, mayonnaise, and foods containing trans fats.

In a perfect world you would never eat the empty calories and chemicals of processed foods. But for most of us, that would be too rigid and unrealistic. As a general rule, eat processed and refined products as sparingly as you possibly can.

A Note About Alcohol

Research has shown that moderate drinking is good for your heart and cardiovascular system. However, alcoholic drinks also have lots of calories which can lead to increased weight (and we know what that does). And if drinking is a problem in your life, do not use the health benefits of limited amounts as an excuse to overindulge.

Among other things, heavy drinking can causes inflammation of the liver, stomach, pancreas, intestines, and esophagus.

In the United States, one drink is 12 ounces of beer, 5 ounces of wine, or 1½ ounces of hard liquor. The latest recommendations for alcohol consumption are for women to have no more than one drink per day, and that men have no more than two drinks per day. These guidelines are from the U.S. Department of Agriculture and the Food and Drug Administration's Dietary Guidelines for Americans.

Fiber, Sugar, and Cholesterol

Now that you have looked at the seven principles of the anti-inflammation diet, you may be asking: "What about fiber? Sugar? Cholesterol?" The answer is that guidelines for them are incorporated into the seven principles.

A Note About Fiber

Fiber is part of all healthy diets. Adults should get at least the minimum recommended amount of 20 to 35 grams of dietary fiber per day (see Chapter 8). Grains, fruits, and vegetables are all healthy sources of fiber. If you follow all of the seven principles of the anti-inflammation diet, you will get plenty of nutrient-rich fiber in your diet.

A Note About Sugar

Eating refined sugar causes quick and strong increases in blood sugar, which, over time, can be damaging to your health. In fact, too much sugar has been linked to an increased risk of diabetes and heart disease. If you follow the seven principles covered in this chapter you will be cutting way back on refined sugars, and you will be getting sugar naturally from the fruits, vegetables, and grains you eat.

A Note About Cholesterol

Cholesterol has a not-always-deserved bad reputation. It is actually an important molecule that has many key roles in our bodies' chemistries. Cholesterol is carried in the bloodstream as lipoproteins. Low-density lipoprotein (LDL) cholesterol is the bad cholesterol because elevated levels go hand and hand with high risk of heart disease. High-density lipoprotein (HDL) cholesterol is the good cholesterol because high levels are associated with less coronary disease.

A diet high in saturated fats tends to be a guilty party when LDL levels are high. Eating foods with cholesterol actually has much less impact on high levels of LDL or low levels of HDL than the type of fat you eat. In addition, there are factors beyond diet, such as genetic makeup, that control the level of LDL (bad) cholesterol. Once again, if you follow the seven principles covered in this chapter, particularly if you cut saturated and trans fats out of your diet, you will be on the right track.

The Least You Need to Know

- Eat a variety of foods to maintain health.

- Cut out bad fats, including saturated fats and trans fatty acids.

- Eat more omega-3s, other healthy fats, lean proteins, grains, fruits, and vegetables.

- Cut out processed and refined foods.

Chapter 5

How the Anti-Inflammation Diet Works

In This Chapter

- ◆ Understand the Healthy Eating Pyramid
- ◆ Connect the pyramid to the seven principles of healthy eating
- ◆ Understand the importance of antioxidant-rich carbs and phytochemicals in your diet
- ◆ Learn about trigger and inflammatory foods and why you should avoid them
- ◆ Recipes for an anti-inflammation diet

The seven principles of the anti-inflammation diet (which were presented in Chapter 4) draw on the best available research about diet and inflammation. The diet emphasizes cutting down on foods that foster inflammation, and stepping up those that fight inflammation. It also emphasizes the importance of losing any excess fat, which contributes to inflammation.

The first principle of the anti-inflammation diet is to eat a well-balanced variety of wholesome foods. We believe that the best approach to accomplish this is to follow the advice of Dr. Walter Willett and his colleagues at the Harvard School of Public Health (HSPH). They have developed the Healthy Eating Pyramid, which is different than the U.S. Department of Agriculture's pyramid (www.mypyramid.gov) and is based on sound scientific research conducted at HSPH and other highly respected research centers.

The Healthy Eating Pyramid

Notice that Dr. Willett's approach is based on the premise that foods near the base of the model are health-promoting. They are the foundation of the diet, and should be eaten frequently. Those on the higher levels of the pyramid should be eaten sparingly.

In other words, the farther a food type is from the base, the more harmful it is for you, and this holds true for its impact on inflammation. The foods on the detached peak are the worst. A good rule of thumb is to think of these foods as being for special occasions only.

How to Climb the Pyramid

The pyramid's food guidelines include several levels. The following text describes each level in detail:

The First Level

The base, also referred to as the first level, of the Healthy Eating Pyramid is daily exercise and weight control, which greatly promotes health and prevents metabolic syndrome.

The Second Level

◆ Whole-grain foods—These are healthy carbohydrates, which your body needs for energy. Eat them at most meals.

◆ Plant oils—Because most people get one third or more of their calories from fats, they are on the first floor of the pyramid. However, the fats you eat must be health promoters. Stay away from animal fats and palm, palm kernel, and coconut oils.

The Third Level

◆ Vegetables (in abundance daily) and Fruits (2–3 times daily)—As we mentioned previously, men should eat nine servings of fruits and vegetables a day and women should eat seven servings.

The Fourth Level

◆ Nuts and legumes (1–3 times daily)—Nuts and legumes are excellent sources of protein, fiber, vitamins, and minerals.

The Fifth Level

◆ Fish, poultry, and eggs (0–2 times daily)—These are important sources of lean protein, but you do not have to eat them every day if you eat other wholesome sources of protein.

The Sixth Level

◆ Dairy or calcium supplement (1–2 times)—Dairy products are great sources of protein but can contain a lot of saturated fat. The developers of the HSPH pyramid point out that three glasses of whole milk have as much saturated fat as 13 strips of cooked bacon! Stick to no-fat or low-fat dairy products. Or get your calcium from other sources. For example, broccoli and soybeans are loaded with calcium, and there are many other plant foods chock-full of the nutrient.

The Detached Peak: Step Carefully

Stay away from these foods as much as possible:

◆ Red meat and butter—These are on the peak of the Healthy Eating Pyramid because they contain lots of saturated fat.

◆ White rice, white bread, potato, white pasta, soda, and sweets—These are also at the top of the Healthy Eating Pyramid because they can cause "fast and furious increases in blood sugar that can lead to weight gain, diabetes, heart disease, and other chronic disorders," according to Dr. Willett. Notice that the well-loved standby, potatoes, are included in these stay-away-from foods.

 InflamWise

The beloved potato, naked (without butter or any other topping), has a high glycemic index (GI). In other words, potatoes cause a rapid, strong rise in blood sugar. Over time, these surges may damage the cells that produce the hormone insulin.

In addition, Dr. Willett and his colleagues also recommend the following:

◆ Take a multivitamin daily. A daily multivitamin, multimineral supplement is a "nutritional backup." The developers of the Healthy Eating Pyramid remind us that taking a vitamin/mineral supplement can't replace healthy eating, or make up for unhealthy eating. However, "it can fill in the nutrient holes that may sometimes affect even the most careful eaters," according to Dr. Willett.

◆ Drink alcohol only in moderation. Research has found that an alcoholic drink a day lowers the risk of heart disease. However, moderation is key. The developers of the pyramid say, "For men, a good balance point is one to two drinks a day. For women, it's at most one drink a day."

The Healthy Eating Pyramid and the Anti-Inflammation Diet

The anti-inflammation diet incorporates the building blocks of the Healthy Eating Pyramid. Here is how:

1. Eat a well-balanced variety of wholesome foods

This means eating a balance of foods from all levels of the pyramid up to the peak, which can include some red meat, white rice, white pasta, and potatoes.

2. Eat only unsaturated fats

   Choose oils listed at the base of the pyramid: olive, canola, soy, corn, sunflower, peanut, and other vegetable oils. But do not eat palm, palm kernel, or coconut oil.

3. Eat one good source of omega-3 fatty acids every day

   Okay, we added this one. Even though Dr. Willett suggests in his book *Eat, Drink, and Be Healthy* that you should eat one good source of omega-3 fatty acids a day, he didn't specifically include them in the Healthy Eating Pyramid. We believe that getting enough omega-3s in your diet plays such an important role in preventing inflammation that we have made it Principle #3. In addition, eat coldwater fish such as salmon at least twice a week.

4. Eat a lot of whole grains

   Whole grains are on the base of the pyramid. Eat them at most meals.

5. Eat healthy sources of protein

   Get your protein from nuts, legumes, fish, poultry, and eggs.

6. Eat plenty of fruits and vegetables

   Need we say more?

7. Eliminate refined and processed foods as much as possible

   Refined foods are in the detached peak along with red meat and butter. Eat sparingly if at all.

Summing Up

Here is a summary of the seven steps as they relate to the pyramid:

◆ Eat a balanced and varied diet.

◆ Eat whole grains at most meals.

◆ If you are a woman, aim to eat seven or more servings of fruits and vegetables. If you are a man, aim to eat nine or more servings.

◆ Use only healthful fats.

◆ Eat nuts and/or legumes at least once—three times during the day is better.

◆ If you are getting enough protein it is okay to cut out fish, poultry, and eggs. Regardless, eat no more than two servings a day.

◆ Eat low-fat dairy foods no more than two times.

◆ Eat one good source of omega-3 fatty acids every day.

◆ Drink alcohol only in moderation.

◆ Take a daily multivitamin.

Who Should Practice the Anti-Inflammation Diet

The anti-inflammation diet is a lifelong approach to nutrition that everyone should follow regardless of their age. At the same time, some people are particularly at risk for inflammatory conditions and should make sure to follow the diet's guidelines. This applies to you if any of the following are true:

◆ You have a high CRP level.

◆ You have any indication of heart disease such as high cholesterol, high blood pressure, and so on.

◆ You have diabetes or a doctor has told you that you could develop diabetes.

◆ You have an inherited risk of heart disease, stroke, diabetes, Alzheimer's disease, asthma, and so on.

◆ You have arthritis.

◆ You have an autoimmune disorder such as asthma, rheumatoid arthritis, or lupus.

◆ You have dental problems—gum disease or periodontal disease.

◆ You have any of the diseases ending in "-itis."

Maintaining an anti-inflammatory lifestyle is important to maximize the effectiveness of the diet.

A Key to Success: Maintain a Healthy Weight

Although the anti-inflammation diet is not a diet to lose pounds, controlling body weight is an important weapon in the arsenal to fight inflammation.

Your daily calorie needs depend on how much you weigh and how active you are. There are a number of ways to calculate the number of calories you need per day to maintain your present weight. On the web, the American Cancer Society offers a quick and easy calculator that takes into consideration your current weight, sex, and activity level. Check the Internet resource section in this book, Appendix C, for more information.

The rule about weight control is the old standby: calories in = calories out. This understanding of weight maintenance has not changed even though it has been rigorously studied. If the amount of calories you take in equals the amount that you spend through daily activity, your weight will remain the same. If the amount of calories you take in is more than you spend, you will gain weight. The opposite is true if you take in less than you spend. The path to weight loss is eating less and exercising more, or both.

Whether you weigh 115 or 215, a pound of body weight is equal to 3,500 calories. If you eat 500 fewer calories per day than the amount of calories you need, you will lose 1 pound per week. You could also perform enough exercise to equal another 500 calories per day—such as exercising on an elliptical machine for 30 minutes—and you will lose 2 pounds.

We cover this topic with more detail in Chapter 17.

The Anti-Inflammation Diet Includes Antioxidant-Rich Carbs

One of the advantages of following the anti-inflammation approach to nutrition is that your diet will be full of healthful unrefined carbohydrates and not empty calories. A diet full of colorful fruits, vegetables, and whole grains supplies a range of important *antioxidants*.

Antioxidant-rich carbohydrates act by blocking "free radicals," which can contribute to silent inflammation. In contrast, the carbohydrates in sugary foods are usually low in antioxidants and contain harmful fats. They also cause overweight and obesity. The exception is dark chocolate, which is rich in antioxidants (but high in calories).

def•i•ni•tion

An **antioxidant** is any substance that reduces damage due to oxygen (oxidative damage) such as that caused by free radicals. Free radicals are highly reactive chemicals that change chemical structures. Well-known antioxidants include vitamin C, vitamin E, and beta carotene (which is converted to vitamin A), all capable of counteracting the damaging effects of oxidation.

The Anti-Inflammation Diet Promotes Omega-3 Fatty Acids

As we discuss in Chapter 4, omega-3 fatty acids are one of the most important weapons against inflammation. They are so important that the American Heart Association recommends eating fish (particularly fatty fish) at least two times a week.

> **What the Experts Say**
>
> *Fish is a good source of protein and doesn't have the high saturated fat that fatty meat products do. Fatty fish like mackerel, lake trout, herring, sardines, albacore tuna, and salmon are high in two kinds of omega-3 fatty acids, eicosapentaenoic acid (EPA) and docosahexaenoic acid (DHA).*
>
> —The American Heart Association

AHA also recommends eating tofu and other forms of soybeans, canola, walnut and flaxseed, and their oils. These contain alpha-linolenic acid (also known as LNA or linolenic acid), which can become omega-3 fatty acid in the body. However, most experts do not think that these sources are as potent or effective as getting omega-3s directly from fatty fish.

Omega-3 supplements are also available. However, if you take more than 3 grams of omega-3 fatty acids a day, it is very important to discuss this with your doctor.

Phytochemicals

Another advantage of following the anti-inflammation diet is that you will consume a lot of phytochemicals. A phytochemical is a natural compound found in plant foods.

Research suggests that phytochemicals, working together with nutrients found in fruits, vegetables, and nuts, may help slow inflammation and related diseases. These protective plant compounds are an emerging area of nutrition and health, with new research reported every day.

> **Did You Know?**
>
> More than 900 different phytochemicals have been found in plant foods, and more are being discovered each year.

Fruits and vegetables that are bright colors—yellow, orange, red, green, blue, and purple—usually contain the most phytochemicals and the most nutrients.

Eating lots of fruits, vegetables, whole grains, soy, and nuts will give you a lot of phytochemicals in your diet. Blueberries, strawberries, and other berries are great choices. In addition, apples and red onions are excellent sources of quercetin, which has strong anti-inflammatory properties.

One of the best-known groups of phytochemicals is the carotenoids, the pigments that give fruits and vegetables their bright colors. One carotenoid, beta-carotene, is eventually converted by the body into vitamin A. This phytochemical is found abundantly in carrots, spinach, and sweet potatoes.

Another type of carotenoid is called lycopene, which is found abundantly in processed tomato products such as tomato sauce and ketchup. It is thought to reduce the risk of prostate cancer.

Avoid Eating Trigger Foods

If you have food allergies or intolerances, they can cause inflammatory reactions. Eliminating the foods that trigger these conditions from your diet can bring tremendous relief. Here is a quick overview.

There are two types of food triggers: allergies and intolerances. They are not the same thing, but they both cause inflammation. If you have a food allergy your immune system reacts to a certain food protein that it thinks is poisonous. The most common form of food allergy occurs when your body creates immunoglobulin E (IgE) *antibodies* to the food you are allergic to. When these IgE antibodies react with the food, chemicals cause inflammation, hives, asthma, or other symptoms of an allergy.

def•i•ni•tion

An **antibody** is special protein that your body makes to defend you against bacteria, viruses, and other foreign materials. Individual antibodies attack and disable specific foreign materials.

Although it is possible to be allergic to any food, such as fruits, vegetables, and meats, there are eight foods that account for 90 percent of all food-allergic reactions. They are: milk; eggs; peanuts; tree nuts such as walnuts and cashews; fish; crustacean shellfish; soybeans; and wheat.

Beginning January 1, 2006, the Food and Drug Administration (FDA) required food labels to clearly state if products contain any proteins from these eight major allergenic foods.

Food intolerances do not involve the immune system. A food intolerance is a problem with the body's metabolism. Milk lactose and wheat gluten are common triggers. If you are sensitive to these foods, your symptoms can include gas, bloating, and abdominal pain.

When you eat the anti-inflammation way, you will be taking in a lot of omega-3s, antioxidant-rich carbs, and phytochemicals.

Eliminate Inflammatory Foods

Some foods trigger inflammation. For example, foods high in omega-6s produce inflammation. Trans fats also trigger inflammation. Here is a summary of the harmful foods you should eliminate from your diet:

- ◆ Animal fats (if you do eat red meat, choose grass-fed, low-fat buffalo/bison)
- ◆ Saturated fats and any products that contain saturated fats
- ◆ Trans fats and any products that contain trans fats
- ◆ Fried foods
- ◆ Some plant oils, such as palm and coconut, and any products that contain them
- ◆ Drinks with added sugar, including some fruit juices
- ◆ Refined sugar and any products that contain any of the many forms of sugar
- ◆ Refined flour and any products that contain refined flour
- ◆ Refined grains

Recipes

One-Pot Meals

Cookbook writer Elizabeth Yarnell has developed a new, quick and healthy approach to cooking an entire meal in one pot. She calls her technique "Glorious One-Pot Meals." Each recipe contains an entrée, grains, and vegetable side dishes for a complete meal with minimal preparation or clean-up.

Yarnell's method is unique in that it allows ingredients to retain their shape and integrity throughout the cooking process, unlike other one-pot meal methods such as crock-pot stews, casseroles, and stir-fries. The following recipe is from her book, *Glorious One-Pot Meals* (Pomegranate Consulting, 2005).

Yarnell's recipes take under half an hour to prepare and less than 1 hour in the oven. The infusion cooking method packs each ingredient with flavor without any disintegration. Food emerges whole and intact from the pot to your mouth. Each recipe bakes in a 2-quart enamel-coated Dutch oven and feeds two adults. Enamel cast-iron Dutch ovens distribute heat evenly on all sides. To serve four, use at least a 4-quart Dutch oven and double the recipe. Larger meals may increase the baking time. Below is one of Yarnell's recipes for salmon.

Salmon with Capers

¼ cup raw barley

½–¾ lb. salmon fillets

Salt and pepper to taste

4 cloves garlic, chopped

1 tsp. capers

½ cup white wine

4 oz. Italian roasted red peppers, cut in pieces

1 head broccoli

Note: Italian roasted red peppers are sold by the jar and packed in olive oil. Be sure to use wild salmon and not farm-raised.

Preheat oven to 450°. Pour barley in a strainer and rinse in cold water. In a small bowl, mix barley with ½ cup water, lightly salt and pepper, and set aside.

Spray inside of 2-quart Dutch oven and lid with olive oil. Place salmon in bottom of pot, skin side down if with skin. Spray fillets lightly with olive oil. Season with salt and pepper to taste. Sprinkle with garlic and capers. Pour half of the wine over the fish. Top with roasted red peppers.

Pour barley over top. Add the broccoli florets and arrange to fit inside pot. Pour rest of wine over all.

Cover and bake for 45 minutes.

Salad Dressings

Both of these salad dressings are great with any combination of greens and fresh vegetables.

Avocado Salad Dressing

¼ seedless cucumber, finely diced

1 ripe avocado, mashed

1 tomato, finely diced

¼ tsp. onion powder

¼ tsp. garlic powder

1 TB. chopped onion or scallion

½ tsp. chicken bouillon powder

1 TB. lemon juice

1 tsp. honey or other sweetener

1 TB. light mayonnaise

Salt to taste

Make this right before you serve it as the avocado turns brown quickly. Blend all ingredients except the cucumber, tomato, and onion. Add water to desired thickness. Stir in the diced cucumber, tomato, and onion and serve.

Japanese Carrot Salad Dressing

1 small carrot; peeled and shredded

2 TB. Mirin (a Japanese cooking wine)

2 TB. rice vinegar or cider vinegar

1 TB. soy sauce

½ tsp. dark sesame oil

1 TB. grated fresh ginger root

3 oz. silken tofu (this will thicken it up)

Blend all ingredients.

Black Soybean Salad

Try something different: a salad made with black soybeans, found at your local health-food store.

1 (16-oz.) can black soybeans, drained and rinsed

1 cup canned or cooked corn kernels, drained

1 cup sliced celery

½ cup diced sweet red peppers

½ cup green peppers

¼ cup sliced green onions

¼ cup ripe olives

2 TB. pickled hot yellow peppers, seeded and diced

¼ cup soybean oil (vegetable oil)

¼ cup white wine vinegar

¾ tsp. salt

½ tsp. chili powder

Freshly ground pepper to taste

Combine soybeans, corn, celery, sweet peppers, green onions, olives, and hot peppers in a large bowl; toss to mix. Combine remaining ingredients in a small bowl and whisk to blend all ingredients. Pour dressing over soybean mixture. Marinate at least 1 hour.

Courtesy of the United Soy Board.

Spaghetti with Turkey Meat Sauce

A health-promoting version of an old standby.

1 lb. ground turkey, lean

1 (28-oz.) can tomatoes, cut up

1 cup green pepper, finely chopped

1 cup onion, finely chopped

2 cloves garlic, minced

1 tsp. dried oregano, crushed

1 tsp. black pepper

1 lb. whole-grain spaghetti noodles, uncooked

Cooking spray

Coat large skillet with nonstick spray. Preheat over high heat. Add turkey and cook, stirring occasionally, for 5 minutes. Drain and discard fat. Stir in tomatoes with juice, green pepper, onion, garlic, oregano, and black pepper. Bring to boil. Reduce heat and simmer covered for 15 minutes, stirring occasionally. Remove cover and simmer for another 15 minutes. (For creamier sauce, give sauce a whirl in blender or food processor.)

Meanwhile, cook spaghetti in unsalted water. Drain well. Serve sauce over spaghetti noodles.

From Heart Health Recipes *(National Heart, Lung, and Blood Institute)*.

Green Tea Slushie

Green tea is a popular antioxidant. The ingredient that separates this treat from other iced green tea drinks is powdered green tea, which can be found in health food or specialty tea stores.

1 tsp. powdered green tea   **¾ cup low-fat or skim milk**

1 TB. brown sugar   **1 cup ice**

⅛ tsp. vanilla

Blend the tea, sugar, vanilla, and milk. Put ice in last and blend to desired consistency. Add more sugar if needed.

The Least You Need to Know

◆ The base of the Healthy Eating Pyramid begins with exercise and weight control.

◆ Eat foods on the higher levels of the pyramid only on special occasions.

◆ Follow the anti-inflammation diet to get ample phytochemicals and antioxidants.

◆ Avoid food triggers, which can cause inflammation.

Chapter 6

Putting It into Action: Fats

In This Chapter

- ◆ Differentiate good fats from harmful fats
- ◆ Learn how to spot trans fats
- ◆ How to choose olive oils
- ◆ See the myths and realities of canola oil
- ◆ Thinking fruit
- ◆ Recipes for an anti-inflammation diet

Inflammatory health problems, such as heart disease or arthritis, are not a consequence of how much fat you eat, but what type. Research has shown that the amount of fat in your diet does not cause health conditions. However, if you eat harmful fats—saturated and trans fats—you are far more likely to develop an inflammatory disease.

The key is to substitute good fats for harmful fats. That is why Principle #2 of the anti-inflammation diet is to eat only unsaturated fats.

Eat Only Good Fats

Substituting good fats for saturated and trans fats is easier than it sounds. If you've ever dipped a chunk of bread into a pool of fragrant olive oil, you know what we mean.

Good and harmful fats are listed in this table.

Dietary Fats

Type of Fat	Main Source	State at Room Temperature
Good Fats		
Monounsaturated	Olives, olive oil, canola oil, peanut oil, walnut oil, most other nut oils, avocados	Liquid
Polyunsaturated	Corn, soybean, safflower, cottonseed oil, fish oil	Liquid
Harmful Fats		
Saturated	Animal products, such as whole milk, butter, cheese, ice cream, red meat; plant products, such as chocolate, coconuts, coconut milk, coconut oil, palm oil	Solid
Trans	Many margarines, soft vegetable shortening, partially hydrogenated vegetable oil, many deep-fried foods, many fast foods, many commercial baked goods	Solid

The Worst of the Lot: Trans Fats

We'll say it again: trans fats are the gang leaders when it comes to inflammation. However, more and more alternatives are becoming available for those of us who want to stay away from them.

Many regulators and food producers have responded to consumers and worked to eliminate trans fats in products. For example, in 2005, the New York City Department of Health and Mental Hygiene asked city restaurateurs and food suppliers to voluntarily eliminate trans fats from their kitchens. Commissioner Dr. Thomas R. Frieden said:

> To help combat heart disease, the number-one killer in New York City, we are asking restaurants to voluntarily make an oil change and remove artificial trans fat from their kitchens. We are also urging food suppliers to provide products that are trans-fat-free.

That is quite a statement for a city government official to make.

Great progress has been made across industry. Even Crisco, the definitive trans fat product, now sells a trans-fat-free version. (Original Crisco, with 4 grams of trans fats per tablespoon, is still available.) And Girl Scouts are now selling trans-fat-free Thin Mints. (Girl Scouts of the USA promises to eliminate trans fats from more cookies.)

Many food manufacturers and supermarket chains have recently replaced trans fats with more healthful substitutes in their products. "Trans-fat-free" labels are showing up on every aisle of the grocery store. For example, Promise and Olivio are trans-fat-free. And Frito-Lay now uses trans-fat-free oils for making Doritos and other snacks.

However, others "are still frying french fries, chicken nuggets, and other fast foods in trans-fat-laden, heart-attack-inducing partially hydrogenated oils," according to a survey conducted by the Center for Science in the Public Interest (CSPI).

Trans fat labeling on packaged foods became mandatory on January 1, 2006. In an examination of the issue, CSPI found that the looming deadline was a powerful incentive for supermarkets and food manufacturers to switch to healthier oils. However, CSPI also found that the lack of similar requirements for restaurant chains means that they still serve trans-fat-laden foods.

However, here is a summary of restaurants that CSPI did find safe to patronize:

- Au Bon Pain, a 220-location café chain based in Boston, has eliminated trans fat from all of its cookies, bagels, and muffins, and uses a nonhydrogenated margarine.

- Jason's Deli, a 137-outlet sandwich and salad chain, has stopped using partially hydrogenated oils in all of its products.

- Panera Bread, a 773-outlet café chain that was formerly part of Au Bon Pain, has removed all trans fats from its menu.

- California Pizza Kitchen has removed trans fats from deep-fried foods and is working on eliminating it from all other foods.

- Ruby Tuesday, with some 700 table-service restaurants around the country, now deep fries in heart-healthy canola oil, though its suppliers still fry some items in partially hydrogenated oil.

- Chik-fil-A fries in peanut oil in its outlets, though its suppliers also par-fry french fries in partially hydrogenated oil.

In addition, according to CSPI:

- Kraft has eliminated most or all trans fat from Triscuts, Wheat Thins, Chips Ahoy, Mallomars, Reduced Fat Oreos, Oreos, Boca products, Honey Maid low-fat Cinnamon Grahams, SnackWell's Cracked Pepper crackers, and other products.

- Gorton's has replaced partially hydrogenated oils with healthier oils in its entire line of fish sticks and fillets.

- George Weston Bakeries plans to eliminate trans fat in all Entenmann's and Freihofer cake and danish products.

- McCain now uses canola oil for all of its grocery and retail frozen potatoes and one line of its food-service french fries.

- Rich Products has reformulated more than 500 products, mostly targeted for the food service industry, to remove trans fat.

- Supermarket chains are also making progress, according to CSPI. Whole Foods has never sold foods with partially hydrogenated oil, and 9 of 11 chains that responded to CSPI's queries say they have already made changes or plan to do so for their store-brand products. Wegman's, which has more than 70 stores in New

York, Pennsylvania, New Jersey, Virginia, and Maryland, has been making gradual changes for years; Raley's, which owns and operates 138 stores in California, Nevada, and New Mexico, and Giant chains, which has 202 supermarkets in Maryland, Virginia, Delaware, New Jersey, and Washington, D.C., have asked suppliers to make changes and have switched to trans-fat-free McCain for store-brand frozen french fries.

Although progress has been made, trans fats are still lurking out there. Here is what you should watch out for:

◆ If hydrogenated oil, partially hydrogenated oil, or vegetable shortening appear on the ingredients list of a product, stay away.

◆ A lot of margarines contain trans fats: stick margarine is worse than soft margarine. For example, Land O'Lakes stick margarine has 2.5 grams of trans fats per serving. Dip bread in flavored olive oil instead of margarine.

◆ Choose Benecol, Take Control, or other margarine-like spreads. They contain plant derivatives that have been shown to lower LDL cholesterol levels by 10 to 14 percent. They have an ingredient called sitostanol, an ingredient found in plants that lowers cholesterol absorption.

◆ Try not to buy commercially prepared baked goods and fast foods unless you have read the ingredients list and are sure that they do not include trans fats (partially hydrogenated oil or vegetable shortening).

◆ When foods containing trans fats can't be avoided, choose products that list them near the end of the ingredient list.

◆ Stay away from deep-fried foods.

More Caution

The best approach is to cut french fries, chips, pies, pizza, and cookies from your diet. Some nutritionists recommend limiting fat to no greater than 30 percent of daily calories and saturated fat to no more than 10 percent of daily calories. (Less is better.) This table lists the amount of fat that provides 30 percent of calories for diets at different total daily calorie levels.

Total Calories	Total Fat (g)	Saturated Fat (g)
Per Day	*30% of Calories*	*10% of Calories*
1,600	53	18
2,000	65	20
2,200	73	24
2,500	80	25
2,800	93	31

Values for 2,000 and 2,500 calories are rounded to the nearest 5 g.
Source: U.S. Department of Agriculture and Department of Health and Human Services (2000).

Choose Good Oils

The top fat that you should use to replace harmful fats is olive oil. Canola oil is second in line. You also might want to consider flaxseed and nut oils, because they contain the inflammation-fighting omega-3s.

Olive Oil

Olive oils are an important part of the anti-inflammation arsenal, so it is important to know how to choose and keep them. Labeling of olive oils can be confusing and deceptive. For example, bottles labeled "Made in Italy" may mean that the olives are grown in Spain and "light oils" are light in color but not in calories or fat. They also lack the rich flavor of darker oil.

The best olive oils come from countries on the Mediterranean and Adriatic (Italy, Greece, Spain, and so on). The International Olive Oil Council (IOOC) sets complicated standards for oils. The labels you should look for in stores, however, show an oil's grade:

◆ The highest-quality olive oil is extra-virgin. If you can afford it, this should be your first choice. It comes from the first pressing of the olives, contains no more than 0.8 percent acidity, and does not include any refined oil.

◆ Virgin olive oil has an acidity less than 2 percent, and is judged to have a good taste. There can be no refined oil in virgin olive oil.

- Olive oil is a blend of virgin oil and refined virgin oil, containing at most 1 percent acidity. It commonly lacks a strong flavor.

- After oils are extracted from olives, there is a solid substance left over called pomace, which still contains a small quantity of oil. Olive-pomace oil is a blend of oil from the pomace and other olive oils.

InflamWarnings

Flavored olive oils and dressings are delicious, but be careful. Unless they are going to be served immediately, never put anything in oils that contains water, including garlic, lemon peel, fresh peppers, fresh herbs, and spices. The water in such items can breed bacteria, including botulism.

Labels May Not Mean What They Say

When labels on olive oils say "Imported from Italy," it may mean just that. The oil is imported from Italy but grown in Spain or somewhere else. Spain is the leading producer of olives with more than 40 percent of world production, followed by Italy and Greece. Much of the Spanish crop is exported to Italy, where it is distributed or repackaged for sale abroad as Italian olive oil.

Here are some other clever and confusing wordings to look out for on olive oil labels:

- "100% Pure Olive Oil" is actually low quality. Better grades have "virgin" on the label.

- "Made from refined olive oils" actually means that the contents were chemically produced.

- "Lite olive oil" does not mean a low fat content. It means a lighter color. All olive oil has 120 calories per tablespoon.

- "From hand-picked olives" is meaningless. There is no evidence that hand-picking olives is better than the common tree-shaking method.

Did You Know?

For high-quality oils, choose expeller-pressed, unrefined oils. They retain most of their nutrients, flavor, aroma, and color. In addition, cooking oils can become rancid when exposed to heat, light, and oxygen. Purchase olive oil sold in cans or dark bottles. If using a transparent bottle, store it in a dark, cool place.

Canola Oil

Canola oil is another monounsaturated oil that, like olive oil, can fight inflammation when it is used in place of saturated fats. However, its formulation is not quite as favorable as olive oil.

Canola oil comes from the rapeseed plant, which is part of the mustard family of plants. Using canola oil as a food is controversial. Reports on the dangers of rapeseed oil are rampant on the Internet, mostly stemming from an article, "Blindness, Mad Cow Disease and Canola Oil," by John Thomas, which appeared in *Perceptions* magazine, March/April 1996.

Others think canola oil is highly beneficial because it is a monounsaturated oil, and it contains erucic acid, which was the magic ingredient in Lorenzo's oil, the subject of a popular movie about a cure for a genetic illness, adrenoleukodystrophy.

Here are some of the myths and realities about canola oil:

- ◆ Canola oil is rumored to be genetically engineered. In fact, its development predated genetic engineering by almost 20 years. However, some forms of canola are now genetically engineered. If this is a concern, buy only organic canola oil.

- ◆ It is rumored to contain the devilish trans fats. Canola oil that has not been purposely treated to contain trans fatty acids will not have significant amounts of them.

- ◆ Canola oil has a reputation as a biopesticide, which is a natural pesticide that is less toxic than conventional pesticides. Canola, along with other vegetable oils such as soybean oil, is classified as a biopesticide, which means that its action is based on biological effects, not on chemical poisons. It suffocates pests; it does not poison them.

- ◆ Canola oil is a member of the mustard plant family. However, it has no relationship to mustard gas, which received its name because of the color of the gas and the sulfur odor.

- ◆ Just because canola oil can be used as an industrial oil, such as a lubricant or fuel, does not mean that it is dangerous to consume. Many oils are both industrial and edible oils, depending on how they are prepared. In fact, flaxseed, which is full of healthy omega-3 fatty acids, is used to make linoleum.

- ◆ Canola is rumored to be a toxic weed that insects will not eat. In fact, canola is made from rapeseed and is susceptible to pests that thrive in temperate climates.

Canola oil contains 58 percent monounsaturated fatty acids compared to 72 percent in olive oil. Here is a table that compares the most widely used oils:

Oil	% Saturated	Monounsaturated	Polyunsaturated	ALA
Canola	7	58	29	12
Coconut	87	6	2	0
Corn	13	24	60	1
Olive	13	72	8	1
Palm	50	37	10	0
Peanut	17	49	32	1
Safflower	9	12	74	0
Soybean	16	44	37	7
Sunflower	10	20	66	2

What the Experts Say

It isn't necessary to count fat grams or whip out a calculator to compute percentage of calories from fat. You have better things to do with your time, the payoff is very small, and so far there's no solid evidence for adopting exact numerical goals for total fat intake. It does make sense to know what is in the fats you eat, or plan to eat, so you can make healthy choices.

—Dr. Walter Willett and colleagues, *Eat Drink, and Be Healthy*

Flaxseed Oil

Flaxseed oil, like olive and canola, is highly unsaturated and health-promoting. In fact, flax and its oil have the most concentrated nonfish source of omega-3 fatty acids. For more information about flax and flaxseed, see Chapter 8.

Nut Oils

Nut oils can give delicious flavor to baked goods, salads, sautés, and pastas. Like the nuts from which they're pressed, nut oils are very low in saturated fats. Almonds, hazelnuts, macadamias, pecans, and pistachios are high in monounsaturated fats, which help to lower blood cholesterol.

Walnut oil is rich in polyunsaturates, and also supplies omega-3s. This nutty oil is used extensively in Europe, primarily in salad dressings and baked goods. Once opened, walnut oil should be kept refrigerated and keeps well for up to 2 years under those conditions.

When purchasing nut oils, try to find expeller-pressed oils. These oils are extracted from their seed or nut using a cold process so that the essential fatty acids and vitamins are left in the oil. They are also tastier than refined oils.

Pretend Fats

Fat performs many vital functions in cooking, some of which can be duplicated by other products. Fat substitutes were developed to help people lower their fat intake. They work in different ways, such as retaining the moisture that fats provide or mimicking the texture and feel of fat in the mouth. The product olestra is an artificial fat that is not absorbed by the body. Monoglycerides and diglycerides are parts of vegetable oils that are emulsified with water. They have the same calories as fat, but food producers add them in small enough amounts so that they don't have to list them on nutrition labels, only on ingredients lists.

Although fat substitutes are considered safe by the U.S. Food and Drug Administration (FDA), their long-term effects are not known. However, it may be that within the context of a healthy diet, fat substitutes used appropriately can provide flexibility with diet planning.

Baking? Think Fruit

A variety of fruit purées can replace part or all of the harmful fats in baked goods. Try these for moistness and flavor:

InflamWise

To get approximately ¹/₂ cup of fruit purée, use 4 ounces of fresh berries or juicy fruit or 1 cup of cooked and drained berries or juicy fruit.

- Commercial fruit-based fat substitutes
- Applesauce
- Bananas, mashed
- Pear purée
- Prune purée
- Pumpkin

Although they don't provide the same rich flavor, fruit purées reduce the need for fat because they hold the moisture in baked goods as fats do. And the sugars in fruit help browning. They also tenderize baked goods to some degree, but not as well as fat.

Some baked goods are better suited to using fruit to substitute for fat than others, so you may need to do some experimenting when using fruit purées instead of fat. Purées work best in recipes with other wet ingredients such as honey, milk, molasses, and eggs.

Quick breads, muffins, and dense cakes such as carrot cakes are often good candidates for fruit substitutes. Prune purées are even used successfully in gingerbread and chocolate-flavored baked products such as brownies and cakes. If you cannot eliminate all the fat in a recipe, you often can replace part of it.

> **InflamWise**
>
> To make your own prune purée: Combine 8 ounces (1⅓ cups) pitted prunes and 6 tablespoons hot water in food processor. Process until smooth. Makes 1 cup. Store in refrigerator for 1 to 2 months.

Here are some tips for substituting fruit purées for fat in recipes:

- Replace the desired amount of solid shortening with half as much fat substitute. For instance, if a recipe calls for 1 cup of butter, replace it with ½ cup of fruit purée.

- If a recipe calls for a liquid oil, substitute three fourths as much fruit purée. If the batter seems too dry, add a little more fruit purée.

- You can substitute ⅓ cup of fruit purée for the oil in most boxed cake mixes.

- You may want to start out slowly and replace just part of the fat in a recipe. For example, replace one quarter of the fat with fruit purée, then the next time try half, then three quarters, and so on. If you don't like the taste that results from cutting back that much fat, add some back in. Even adding a tablespoon or two of fat back to a recipe may improve your final product.

- Try low-gluten flours. Taking the fat out of baked goods often makes them tough or rubbery. If you use low-gluten flours such as whole-wheat pastry or oat flour, your baked goods will be lighter. Oat bran, rolled oats, and cornmeal are also low in gluten.

- Minimize mixing. Stirring batter too much toughens the texture of baked goods. Stir only enough to mix well.

◆ Reduce the baking temperature and shorten the baking time. Reduced-fat recipes tend to bake more quickly than those with fat; as a consequence they can be dry. Reduce the oven temperature by 25°F, and take the product out 5 to 10 minutes before baking time.

Recipes

Flax, Apple, and Walnut Muffins

¼ cup flaxseeds, ground	½ tsp. salt
¾ cup whole-wheat flour	1 egg, beaten
¾ cup flour	3 TB. canola oil
½ cup turbinado sugar	½ cup milk
2 tsp. baking powder	1½ cup apples, finely chopped
½ tsp. baking soda	½ cup walnuts, chopped

Preheat oven to 400°F. Grease muffin tins.

Blend flaxseed, flours, sugar, baking powder, baking soda, and salt in a bowl. In a separate bowl, combine egg, oil, and milk. Add the flour mixture to the egg mixture and stir just until blended.

Fold in apples and nuts. Fill muffin tins two thirds full and bake 18 to 20 minutes or until top springs back when touched.

Caper and Olive Oil Tapenade

5 TB. capers	4 garlic cloves
½ cup green olives	½ cup extra-virgin olive oil
2 flat anchovy fillets	

Coarsely chop the ingredients or blend in a food processor. Spoon over slices of French bread or use as a dip.

Pasta with Lemon Olive Oil

Makes 4 servings

Zest of 1 lemon	**½ cup capers**
⅓ cup lemon juice	**2 TB. fresh chopped basil**
½ cup extra-virgin olive oil	**Salt and freshly ground black pepper**
1 or 2 large garlic cloves, minced	**1 lb. whole-grain pasta, prepared**

Grate lemon and combine with lemon juice, olive oil, garlic cloves, capers, basil, and pepper in a large serving bowl. Toss hot cooked pasta with the sauce.

The Least You Need to Know

- Avoid harmful fats, including saturated and trans, whenever possible.

- To replace harmful fats such as margarine, use olive oil or canola oil.

- Try out other oils such as flaxseed and nut oils.

- Also try using fruit purées to replace harmful fats when baking.

Chapter 7

Putting It into Action: Omega-3s

In This Chapter

- ◆ Learn how to get your omega-3s through fatty fish
- ◆ Make sure that the fish you eat is safe
- ◆ See how to get your omega-3s through flax
- ◆ Learn about other sources of omega-3s
- ◆ Recipes for an anti-inflammation diet

Getting a sufficient amount of omega-3 fatty acids in your diet can squelch inflammation and reduce your risk of other health problems such as heart disease, stroke, and inflammation-related cancers. Unfortunately, because of our love of processed and fast foods, most of us get way too much omega-6 fatty acids in our diets, which block the absorption of the small amount of omega-3s that we eat. To compensate, it is important to step up our intake of omega-3s. (To review some of the important facts about omega-3 and omega-6 fatty acids, see Chapter 4.)

It takes some planning and effort to get enough omega-3 fatty acids through the food you eat. The major sources—fatty fish and flaxseed—are not everyday foods. That is why the Principle #3 in the anti-inflammation diet is to eat one good source of omega-3 fatty acids every day. It is important to emphasize the need to add omega-3s to your daily diet.

Fish

The best way to get your omega-3s is to eat fish frequently, particularly salmon and other coldwater fatty fish such as herring, mackerel, anchovies, and sardines. They all have large amounts of omega-3. Larger fatty fish such as tuna have omega-3 in smaller amounts, but when eaten frequently can boost the amount of omega-3s in your diet.

InflamWarnings

When you prepare salmon or other fatty fish, don't fry it! The high temperature damages the good fat. Baking or grilling are great options.

How much fish should you eat? Many studies have found that 500 to 1,000 milligrams of omega-3 fatty acids per day are beneficial. The American Heart Association recommends that adults eat fish, particularly oily fish such as salmon, at least twice a week (3-ounce portions), which averages 500 milligrams a day. The AHA recommends that patients with coronary artery disease take in 1,000 milligrams daily, but never more than 3,000 milligrams.

This table lists common fish by the amount of omega-3 fatty acids that are in one serving (3 ounces):

Omega-3 Fatty Acids in Fish

Over 1 Gram	0.5 to 0.9 Gram	Less than 0.5 Gram
Turbot	Scallops	Carp
Salmon	Crab	Cod
Herring, mackerel, sardines	Shrimp	Grouper
Atlantic bluefish	Sea bass	Halibut (Pacific)
Most shellfish	Snapper	Ocean perch
Pacific oysters	Clams	Mahi Mahi
Squid	Lobster	Orange Roughy

Over 1 Gram	0.5 to 0.9 Gram	Less than 0.5 Gram
Anchovy	Striped bass	Tuna
	Shark	
	Mussels	
	Rainbow trout	

Source: Great Northern Products.

One of the most popular fatty fishes is salmon. However, farmed salmon may contain high levels of toxic substances. PCB (polychlorinated biphenyl) levels may be up to eight times higher in farmed salmon than in wild salmon, and omega-3 content may also be lower than in wild-caught species. (PCBs are chemicals used in industrial processes and may cause cancer in humans.)

A rule of thumb is that the vast majority of Atlantic salmon available on the world market is farmed, whereas the majority of Pacific salmon is wild-caught. Even then, the benefits of eating farmed salmon may still outweigh the risks.

Canned salmon in the U.S. is usually wild and caught in the Pacific, although some farmed salmon is available in canned form. Alaskan salmon is always wild catch.

The good news is the dangers of getting mercury with your fish is generally much lower in salmon then in other fish.

Making Sure Fish Is Safe

Follow these tips for eating fish or shellfish and you will have the benefits of consuming omega-3s while limiting your exposure to harmful substances:

◆ If you can afford it, choose wild salmon over farm-raised salmon. In a landmark study, scientists studied more than 2 metric tons of salmon from the Americas and Europe and found PCBs and other cancer-causing toxins at higher levels in farm-raised salmon than that from the wild.

◆ Remember the larger the fish, the higher the risk of contaminants.

◆ Stay away from shark, swordfish, king mackerel, and tilefish. They have high levels of mercury.

◆ Eat fish that are low in mercury. Five of the most commonly eaten fish that are low in mercury are shrimp, canned light tuna, salmon, pollock, and catfish.

◆ Stay away from albacore ("white") tuna. It has much more mercury than canned light tuna, which is not on the watch list. When you hear warnings about the mercury in tuna, it is albacore tuna that is the concern.

◆ Check advisories about the safety of fish caught in local waters. If no advice is available, eat no more than 6 ounces (one average meal) per week of fish from local waters.

◆ Follow these same recommendations when feeding fish and shellfish to a young child, but serve smaller portions.

Eating Tuna Safely

In the United States, one in six children born every year has been exposed to mercury levels so high that they may have learning disabilities and motor-skill impairment. One of the reasons is America's love of the economical tuna-fish salad. Ironically, although tuna-fish salad may be a dangerous source of mercury, it is also a major source of omega-3 fatty acids in the American diet.

The dangers of mercury in tuna are well known. In fact, in 2004, the Food and Drug Administration and Environmental Protection Agency warned women not to eat a lot of canned tuna during pregnancy because its levels of mercury might harm developing fetuses and nursing babies. And a year earlier the California Attorney General's office had filed suit to force supermarkets, restaurants, and tuna companies to warn customers that tuna (fresh, frozen, and canned), swordfish, and shark sold in their markets contain mercury. The suit was based on the state's Proposition 65, which requires consumer warnings for substances on a toxics list.

Clearly mercury in tuna fish is something to be concerned about. If you are going to eat canned tuna fish to get your omega-3s, the best choice is light tuna rather than albacore, which comes from a larger fish with generally higher levels of mercury. This table provides guidelines on how much canned tuna it is safe to eat, according to the Environmental Protection Agency.

Weight in Pounds	Frequency a Person Can Safely Eat a 6-oz. Can of Tuna	
	White Albacore	*Chunk Light*
11	1 can/4 months	1 can/6 weeks
22	1 can/2 months	1 can/23 days

Weight in Pounds	Frequency a Person Can Safely Eat a 6-oz. Can of Tuna	
	White Albacore	*Chunk Light*
33	1 can/5 weeks	1 can/2 weeks
44	1 can/4 weeks	1 can/12 days
55	1 can/3 weeks	1 can/9 days
66	1 can/3 weeks	1 can/8 days
77	1 can/3 weeks	1 can/week
88	1 can/2 weeks	1 can/6 days
99	1 can/2 weeks	1 can/5 days
110	1 can/12 days	1 can/5 days
121	1 can/11 days	1 can/4 days
132	1 can/10 days	1 can/4 days
143	1 can/9 days	1 can/4 days
154	1 can/9 days	1 can/3 days
165	1 can/8 days	1 can/3 days
176	1 can/week	1 can/3 days
187	1 can/week	1 can/3 days
198	1 can/week	1 can/3 days
209	1 can/6 days	1 can/2 days
220	1 can/6 days	1 can/2 days

Source: Food and Drug Administration test results for mercury and fish, and the Environmental Protection Agency's determination of safe levels of mercury.

By these guidelines, if you weigh 110 pounds you can eat one can of albacore tuna every 12 days or one can of light tuna every 5 days. If you weigh 198 pounds you can eat one can of albacore tuna a week or one can of light tuna every 3 days.

Fish Oil

Fish-oil capsules are the most concentrated form of omega-3 fats. They contain all major omega-3 fats—ALA, EPA, and DHA. However, it is important to know the quality of any capsules you may purchase. The level of polychlorinated biphenyls

(PCBs) and other contaminants in fish-oil supplements can be high. Respectable supplement producers filter the heavy metals and pollutants out of fish oils, which makes them safe.

Consumer Reports (CR) tested 16 top-selling fish-oil supplements and the results were reassuring. All pills contained about the amount of DHA and EPA as they listed on their labels. None were rancid and none contained "significant amounts" of the common contaminants mercury, PCBs, or dioxin. CR recommends purchasing the following fish-oil capsules because they had the best price and were safe and reliable: Kirkland Signature Natural Fish Oil (at Costco) or Member's Mark Omega-3 Fish Oil at Sam's Club.

Fish-oil supplements can have a fishy aftertaste and can cause bad breath and bloating, all of which can be unpleasant. Storing them in the freezer may help. If you are interested in this source of omega-3s, be sure to discuss taking fish-oil supplements with your doctor; combined with other medicines they can cause bleeding problems.

Flax

Flaxseed and its oil are great sources of the omega-3 fatty acid ALA. Flax also contains a significant amount of omega-6, but has around three times more omega-3 as omega-6. Flax adds a pleasant, nutty taste to foods.

Because of their omega-3 content, flax products are flying onto the shelves of supermarkets and specialty stores. For example, omega-3 enriched eggs can now be found in many grocery stores. These eggs contain 8 to 10 times more omega-3 fatty acids than regular eggs.

Here are some tips about adding flax to your diet:

- You should grind whole flaxseeds before using them. Your system cannot digest whole seeds and you will not get the benefit of their omega-3s.

- To keep flax fresh, you should grind it as you need it. Keep milled flax refrigerated in an airtight, opaque container for up to 30 days.

- Milled flax can be purchased or ground at home. It can be added to dough, batters, casseroles, and other cooked foods.

- Flax oil is extracted from whole seeds. It can be used in salad dressings.

- Dietary supplements of flax oil are available. Follow manufacturers' dosages.

◆ Flax can replace fat or eggs in recipes. Three tablespoons of milled flax equals 1 tablespoon of butter, margarine, shortening, or vegetable oil. A tablespoon of milled flax plus 3 tablespoons of water equals one egg.

Walnuts

Walnuts are often referred to as "brain food," because their wrinkled shells look like little brains. They also are good for our brains because they have a high concentration of omega-3 fats. One quarter cup of walnuts contains about 2.3 grams of omega-3s, slightly more than is found in 3 ounces of salmon.

A word of caution: walnuts contain omega-3s but also have high amounts of omega-6, so they are not as beneficial as other sources, such as salmon and flax.

There are three main types of walnuts that are popular: English or Persian walnut, black walnut, and white (or butternut) walnut. English walnuts have a thin shell that is easily broken with a nutcracker. Black walnuts have thicker shells and a stronger flavor. White walnuts are sweeter and oilier, and are more difficult to find.

Other nuts have only trace amounts of omega-3s.

Oils

Extra-virgin olive oil, canola, soybean, and walnut oils all contain omega-3 fatty acids. Ironically, food producers destroy omega-3s in vegetable oils when they hydrogenize them to give them a longer shelf life. And, amazingly, in the process the oils go from health-promoting to health-destroying because they become trans fats.

A word of warning: canola oil contains omega-3, but also has a lot of omega-6 (two to three times as much as the amount of omega-3). However, using canola oil in place of saturated fats is extremely beneficial to health, and is better to use than the following cooking oils: sunflower, safflower, sesame, corn, rice-bran, cottonseed, soy, peanut, grapeseed, and wheat. They are high in omega-6 and low in omega-3.

Poultry, Meats, and Dairy

Animals that graze on grass produce meat with omega-3 fatty acids. Scientists are also working to improve the omega-3 content of beef, chicken, and other meats by feeding them flax. Surprisingly, wild venison and buffalo are both great sources of omega-3s. Buffalo is becoming widely available in supermarkets.

Egg yolks are naturally very high in the omega-6 fatty acid, arachidonic acid. Fortunately, eggs rich in omega-3s are also becoming available from producers who feed their hens flax.

Some studies have shown that organic milk and cheese are good sources of omega-3, particularly compared to regular milk.

Plants

Plant sources of omega-3s include beans and winter squash.

The American Heart Association recommends eating tofu and other forms of soybeans because they contain the omega-3 fatty acid ALA. However, they also warn that the benefit is controversial and may be modest. One cup of soy, navy, or kidney beans provides between 200 and 1,000 milligrams of omega-3s (0.2 to 1.0 grams). A 4-ounce serving of tofu (made from soybeans) provides about 0.4 grams of omega-3s.

For more information on soy products, see Chapter 9.

A cup of winter squash provides about 0.3 grams of omega-3s, equal to the amount you would get in 4 ounces of yellowfin tuna.

Salba is a little-known omega-3 rich supergrain that can now be found in tortilla chips and may soon appear in other products.

Other plants that have small amounts of omega-3s include the following:

- Green leafy vegetables: lettuce, broccoli, kale, purslane, and spinach. (Purslane is a cool, crunchy plant popular in India.)

- Other beans: mungo, kidney, navy, pinto, or lima beans, peas, and split peas. (Mungo beans are particularly high in omega-3 fatty acids. They are sold in many Indian groceries and may be found under the name "urid.")

- Fruits: citrus, melons, and cherries.

New Omega-3 Products

Omega-3 products are popping up all over. They are in pastas, breads, and even tortilla chips. In addition to omega-3-rich eggs, here are some items you might look for on your grocer's shelves:

◆ Omega-3-rich pastas with ingredients such as flaxseed, lentils, and different types of grains.

◆ Omega-3 breads with ingredients like MEG-3, derived from fish oil. The breads contain about 40 mg of EPA and DHA per slice.

◆ Tortilla chips with flax and other ingredients that make them rich in omega-3s.

◆ Omega-3 mayonnaise.

Recipes

Turkey Loaf with Flax

Makes 8 servings

Flax adds to the nutrition of this updated meatloaf.

2 lbs lean ground turkey	**1 tsp. black pepper**
1 cup skim milk	**1 tsp. garlic powder**
½ cup ground flaxseed	**1 tsp. dry mustard**
½ cup dry bread crumbs	**½ tsp. celery salt**
½ cup chopped onion	**¼ tsp. ground thyme**
1 egg, beaten	**¼ cup ketchup**
1 TB. Worcestershire sauce	

In a large bowl, combine turkey, milk, ground flax, crumbs, onion, egg, Worcestershire sauce, pepper, garlic, mustard, celery salt, and thyme. Mix well. Put mixture into a 22×13×8 cm (9"×5"×3") loaf pan. Spread ketchup over top of loaf.

Bake at 350°F for 1 to 1½ hours, until no pink remains. Remove from oven and let stand 5 minutes.

Flax Fried Rice

Makes 2 servings

This is a great recipe for using leftover brown rice.

1 cup long grain brown rice	¾ cup chopped vegetables of your choice (carrots, beans, peas, and so on)
2 cup water	
½ tsp. salt	2 scallions, cut into ¼-inch lengths
2 TB. canola oil	
3 eggs, beaten well	2 TB. soy sauce
½ cup diced cooked lean meat such as chicken	½ tsp. sesame oil
	¼ cup flaxseed, toasted

Prepare rice according to directions and let cool (or use leftover rice). In a large nonstick skillet, over medium heat, heat canola oil. Add eggs and fry until half-cooked. Add rice, breaking up any lumps, stirring quickly to coat the rice. Reduce heat to medium-low; add meat, vegetables, and scallions. Cook, stirring and fluffing rice mixture gently but frequently for about 4 minutes. Add soy sauce, sesame oil, and flaxseed. Reduce heat to low, cover and cook 3 minutes.

To toast flaxseed, spread seeds in small metal pan. Bake at 350°F for 3 to 5 minutes. Stir while toasting.

Granny's Tuna Salad

Be sure to use light and not albacore tuna in this recipe.

1 (6-oz.) can light tuna in water, drained	3 whole walnuts, chopped (about 1 TB.)
1 Granny Smith apple, halved and cored	1 TB. light, fat-free, or canola mayonnaise
	1¼ TB. chopped onion

Place tuna in small bowl and break into small chunks. Finely chop half the apple. Add to tuna with walnuts, mayonnaise and onion. Stir until blended. Thinly slice remaining half of apple and use as garnish.

Cannery Row Soup

Use fish that is low in mercury.

1 clove garlic, minced

3 carrots, cut in thin strips

2 cup celery, sliced

½ cup onion, chopped

¼ cup green peppers, chopped

2 TB. olive oil

1 (28-oz) can whole tomatoes, cut up, with liquid

1 cup clam juice

¼ tsp. dried basil, crushed dried thyme, crushed

⅛ tsp. black pepper

2 lb. fish of your choice

¼ cup fresh parsley, minced

Heat oil in large sauce pan. Sauté garlic, carrots, celery, onion, and green pepper in oil 3 minutes. Add tomatoes, clam juice, basil, thyme, and black pepper. Cover and simmer 10 to 15 minutes or until vegetables are fork tender. Add fish and parsley. Simmer, covered, 5 to 10 minutes more or until fish flakes easily and is opaque. Serve hot.

Baked Trout

2 lb. trout fillet, cut into 6 pieces (any kind of fish can be used)

3 TB. lime juice (about 2 limes)

1 medium tomato, chopped

Half medium onion, chopped

3 TB. cilantro, chopped

½ tsp. olive oil

¼ tsp. black pepper

¼ tsp. salt

¼ tsp. red pepper (optional)

Preheat oven to 350°F. Rinse fish and pat dry. Place in baking dish. In separate dish, mix remaining ingredients together and pour over fish. Bake for 15 to 20 minutes or until fork-tender.

Rockport Fish Chowder

Low-fat milk and clam juice are the secrets to this low-saturated-fat version of chowder.

2 TB. vegetable oil	2 cups bottled clam juice
¾ cup coarsely chopped onion	8 whole peppercorns
½ cup coarsely chopped celery	1 bay leaf
1 cup sliced carrots	1 lb. fresh or frozen (thawed) cod or haddock fillets, cut into ¾-inch cubes
1 potato, raw, peeled and cubed	¼ cup flour
¼ tsp. thyme	3 cups low-fat (1 percent) milk
½ tsp. paprika	1 TB. fresh parsley, chopped

Heat oil in a large saucepan. Add onion and celery and sauté about 3 minutes. Add carrots, potatoes, thyme, paprika, and clam juice. Wrap peppercorns and bay leaves in cheesecloth. Add to pot. Bring to a boil, reduce heat, and simmer 15 minutes.

Add fish and simmer an additional 15 minutes, or until fish flakes easily and is opaque.

Remove fish and vegetables; break fish into chunks. Bring broth to a boil and continue boiling until volume is reduced to 1 cup. Remove bay leaves and peppercorns.

Shake flour and ½ cup milk in a container with a tight-fitting lid until smooth. Add to broth in saucepan with remaining milk. Cook over medium heat, stirring constantly, until mixture boils and is thickened.

Return vegetables and fish chunks to stock and heat thoroughly. Serve hot, sprinkled with chopped parsley.

Fish Veronique

1 lb. white fish

¼ tsp. salt

⅛ tsp. black pepper

¼ cup dry white wine

¼ cup fat-free chicken stock

1 TB. lemon juice

1 TB. soft margarine (trans-fat-free)

2 TB. flour

¾ cup low-fat or skim milk

½ cup seedless grapes

Nonstick cooking spray

Spray 10×6-inch baking dish with nonstick spray. Place fish in pan and sprinkle with salt and pepper. Mix wine, stock, and lemon juice in small bowl and pour over fish. Cover and bake at 350°F for 15 minutes.

Melt margarine in small saucepan. Remove from heat and blend in flour. Gradually add milk and cook over moderately low heat, stirring constantly, until thickened.

Remove fish from oven, and pour liquid from baking dish into "cream" sauce, stirring until blended. Pour sauce over fish and sprinkle with grapes. Broil about 4 inches from heat for 5 minutes or until sauce starts to brown.

Spinach Salad with Oranges and Walnuts

This salad packs an anti-inflammatory punch. To really do it up, serve with salmon.

6 TB. olive oil

¼ cup fresh orange juice

3 green onions, minced

3 TB. unseasoned rice vinegar

1 TB. honey

1 TB. chopped fresh tarragon

1 tsp. grated orange peel

4 oranges

1½ (6-oz.) packages baby spinach

⅔ cup walnuts

Whisk oil, juice, onions, vinegar, honey, tarragon, and orange peel in small bowl. Season with salt and pepper. Peel and section oranges. Combine spinach, half of walnuts, and all orange segments in large bowl with enough dressing to coat. Divide among 6 plates. Sprinkle with walnuts.

Roasted Butternut Squash with Apples

1 lb. butternut squash, peeled, seeded, and cubed

1 tsp. canola oil

1½ tsp. pumpkin-pie spice mix

¼ cup red wine vinegar

¼ cup maple syrup

2 Granny Smith apples, cored and cut into ½-inch cubes

¼ cup chopped pecans

Heat oven to 400°F. Mix squash with oil in a bowl. Add spice mix; toss. Spread squash on an ungreased baking sheet; bake 15 minutes or until squash turns golden brown at the edges. In a bowl, mix vinegar and syrup; pour over squash. Bake 5 minutes. Combine apples, pecans, and squash in a bowl. Let cool; serve.

The Least You Need to Know

◆ Eat a source of omega-3 fatty acids every day.

◆ Make sure that the fish you eat is safe, and know the risk of high mercury levels.

◆ Try getting your omega-3s through flax. (Try some of the flax recipes in this book.)

◆ Also try getting your omega-3s from walnuts, olive oils, animals that graze on grass, beans, winter squash, and other common sources.

◆ Try out some of the new omega-3 products such as enriched eggs and pastas.

8

Putting It into Action: Grains

In This Chapter

- ◆ Whole grains defined
- ◆ Grains as a source of fiber
- ◆ Grains from A to W
- ◆ Recipes for an anti-inflammation diet

Eating a diet rich in *whole-grain foods* can prevent inflammation and delay the development of metabolic syndrome. Hence, they are the fourth principle of the anti-inflammation diet.

What are whole grains and how are they different than other grains? Whole grains and the foods made from them contain all the essential parts of the grain's seed, along with its nutrients. They are carbohydrates that are good for you. Whole grains include amaranth, barley, buckwheat, bulgur, corn, flax, millet, oats, quinoa, rice, sorghum, spelt, triticale, wheat, and wild rice. Many consumers are not aware of the range of wholesome grains available to them.

In this chapter, we explain why whole grains are so good for you. We also give you important information about 15 delicious whole grains for you to try. They will add variety and a high level of nutrition to your diet.

What Are Whole Grains?

Whole grains and the foods made from them contain all the essential parts of the grain's seed or the equivalent. Examples of generally accepted whole-grain foods and flours are amaranth, barley (lightly pearled), brown and colored rice, buckwheat, bulgur, corn and whole cornmeal, emmer, farro, grano (lightly pearled wheat), kamut, millet, oatmeal and whole oats, popcorn, quinoa, sorghum, spelt, teff, triticale, whole rye, whole or cracked wheat, wheat berries, and wild rice.

def•i•ni•tion

The Food and Drug Administration defines **whole-grain foods** as those that contain intact fruit or cereal grains; or ground, cracked, or flaked grains with the same proportion of main ingredients as unmilled grain.

Eating whole grains not only reduces inflammation, but has been shown to reduce the risks of heart disease, stroke, cancer, diabetes, and obesity. Yet even consumers who are aware of the health benefits of whole grains are often unsure of the different varieties, how to find them, and how to prepare them.

In their natural state growing in the fields, whole grains are the entire seed of a plant. The grain is made up of three key parts: the bran, the germ, and the endosperm:

- The bran is the outer covering of the grain, which protects its other two parts of the kernel from the sun, pests, water, and disease. It contains antioxidants, B vitamins, and fiber.

- The germ is the embryo, which can sprout into a new plant. It contains many B vitamins, some protein, minerals, and healthy fats.

- The endosperm is the germ's food supply. It supplies energy to the young plant so it can grow. The endosperm is by far the largest portion of the kernel. It contains starchy carbohydrates, proteins, and small amounts of vitamins and minerals.

Refined grains usually have only the endosperm. Without the bran and germ, about a quarter of a grain's protein is lost, along with key nutrients. Processors enrich refined grains with vitamins and minerals, so they do contribute nutrients, but not with richness that whole grains offer.

Whole grains are enjoyed whole, cracked, split, ground, or milled into flour. If you see the words "whole grain" on a food label, the product is required by the federal government to have virtually the same proportions of bran, germ, and endosperm as the harvested kernel does before it is processed.

Some foods that you may think are whole grains aren't. For example, soybean products and other beans, oily seeds such as sunflower seeds, and roots such as arrowroot do not meet the FDA's definition of whole grain.

In dietary guidelines issued last year, the Food and Drug Administration recommends that people eat at least three whole-grain servings per day, with half of the grains consumed every day being whole grains.

What the Experts Say

Making whole grains a part of your life is also one of the best things you can do to boost metabolism, smooth insulin release, and control blood sugar, not to mention lower your risk of diabetes, cancer, stroke, and heart disease.
—Dr. Connie Gutterson, *The Sonoma Diet*, Meredith Books, 2006.

The FDA's dietary guidelines spurred food makers to step up the use of whole grains in their products. For example, in 2004, General Mills added whole grains to all of the company's breakfast cereals. For example, Cheerios cereals have from 8 to 16 grams of whole grain per serving.

A slick and reliable way to determine whether a product is whole grain is to look for the Whole Grain Stamp, developed by the Whole Grain Council. They are becoming ubiquitous on grain products. The stamps are labeled:

◆ Good Source: identifies a half serving of whole grain

◆ Excellent Source: identifies a full serving of whole grain

◆ 100%/Excellent: identifies a full serving of whole grain and all grains are whole grain.

The stamp features a stylized sheaf of grain on a golden-yellow background with a bold black border. To get the recommended three servings a day of whole grains, eat three whole-grain food products labeled "Excellent Source" or "100%/Excellent," or six products labeled "Good Source."

Words on packages	What they mean
whole grain [name of grain] whole wheat whole [other grain] stoneground whole [grain] brown rice	Contains all parts of the grain.
unbleached flour wheat flour semolina durum wheat organic unbleached flour enriched flour degerminated (on corn meal) bran multigrain (may describe several whole grains or several refined grains, or a mix of both)	Parts of the grain may be missing.

Source: Whole Grain Council.

Fiber

Fiber is a carbohydrate that cannot be digested. It is an important part of your diet because it can make you feel full while limiting how many calories you eat. It also promotes a healthy digestive tract.

Fiber is present in all edible plants, including grains. The fiber in whole grains is generally insoluble, which meant that it does not dissolve in water and often is used to relieve constipation.

Grains vary greatly in the amount of fiber they contain, ranging from 3.5 percent in rice to over 15 percent in barley and bulgur. Many refined grains have the fiber refined out of them. For example, 100 grams of whole-grain wheat flour has 12.2 grams of fiber compared to 2.7 grams in enriched, bleached, all-purpose flour.

def•i•ni•tion

Fiber is the indigestible portion of plant foods that moves food through the digestive system and absorbs water. Grains are great sources of fiber. There are two major types of fiber. Insoluble fiber is simply bulk that changes little as it passes through the body. Soluble fiber, on the other hand, forms a soft gel in solution with water. Most foods provide a mixture of both, but are listed as mostly one or the other. Soluble fiber has been shown to be able to bind bile salts, which may reduce blood cholesterol levels. It also may slow the absorption of glucose from the intestine, thereby requiring less insulin secretion.

How to Add Whole Grains to Your Menus

Here are some tips on adding whole grains to your diet:

◆ Substitute half the white flour with whole-wheat flour in baked goods.

◆ Experiment with other types of whole-grain flour, such as amaranth or spelt.

◆ Add grains to your favorite soup or stew.

◆ When you think "potatoes," think again. In their place try a whole-grain recipe such as the ones at the end of Chapter 3.

◆ Instead of white rice, make pilafs and other ricelike dishes with whole grains. Try the kasha pilaf recipe at the end of this chapter.

◆ Enjoy whole-grain salads.

◆ Try whole-grain breads.

◆ Buy whole-grain pasta.

◆ Look for whole-grain cereals. More and more are appearing on grocery shelves.

◆ Experiment with nontraditional ways of using whole grains. For example, try the Wheat Berry Tapenade recipe at the end of this chapter.

Whole Grains: From A to W

The following sections provide details on 15 nutrition-packed whole grains, which can add delicious variety to your diet.

Amaranth

Amaranth is a superfood masquerading as a tiny grain. An 8,000-year-old plant, it was fed to Aztec runners and warriors to provide large bursts of energy and boost performance.

Amaranth is a rarity among grains. It has a high level of complete protein, and contains lysine, an amino acid missing or negligible in many grains. It also is a good source of dietary fiber and minerals.

Amaranth has a pleasant peppery taste. It has no gluten, so it is popular among people with gluten sensitivities. But it must be mixed with wheat to make leavened breads. Amaranth grains are toasted much like popcorn and mixed with honey or molasses to make a treat called *alegría* in Mexico.

Amaranth products are now available in many varieties such as puffed grain, flour, cereals, bread crumbs, and cookies.

Barley

Barley is one of the oldest cultivated grains. Hulled barley retains many of the whole-grain nutrients but is very slow-cooking. Lightly pearled barley lacks some nutrients but is more easily cooked and digested. The fiber in barley is especially healthy. In fact, it may lower cholesterol even more effectively than oat fiber.

def•i•ni•tion

Gluten is a protein found in flour, which forms during bread making. The gluten forms a network that traps CO_2 created by yeast, giving bread its characteristic texture and air bubbles.

Barley has a rich nutlike flavor. In addition, barley has *gluten*, which gives it a pastalike consistency.

Barley is usually thought of as an addition to soup, but it can be used in hot cereal, salads, and pilafs. It can be mixed with wheat flour to make breads and muffins.

Buckwheat

In the United States buckwheat is primarily known for pancakes. However, it is also the ingredient in soba noodles, popular in Japan, and gaining popularity here. It is also known as kasha, which is a roasted whole-grain buckwheat, popular in Russia and a traditional Sunday dish for many in the United States.

Buckwheat pasta and noodles are a good alternative for you if you are gluten intoler-ant. Technically, buckwheat is not a grain and it is not a form of wheat. It has high levels of an antioxidant called rutin.

Bulgur

Bulgur is a quick-cooking form of whole wheat that has been cleaned, parboiled, dried, ground into particles, and sifted into distinct sizes. It is fiber-rich and has a mild flavor, which makes it popular in dishes such as tabbouleh, a favorite Lebanese salad. Bulgur cooks in about the same time as pasta. This makes it popular for quick side dishes, pilafs, or salads.

Bulgur differs from cracked wheat in that it is precooked. It is ready to eat with mini-mal cooking or, after soaking in water or broth, can be mixed with other ingredients without further cooking. It can be used in recipes calling for rice. But if you are sensi-tive to gluten, stay away from bulgur.

Corn

Today corn is the second most plentiful grain in the world behind rice and ahead of wheat. It is low in fat and calories, and rich in fiber. However, compared to other grains, it is not a great source of nutrients.

Corn is a symbol of American culture. Think Native American heritage. Think the Fourth of July and corn on the cob. Think popped corn at the movies.

Corn sometimes gets a bad rap because people who have relied on corn as the major source of food in their diets develop pellagra, a disease caused by niacin deficiency. Eating corn with beans creates a complementary mix of amino acids, which raises the protein value to humans.

InflamWise

Here are some tips on how to make corn a more nutritious part of your diet:

- When purchasing corn tortillas, purchase those that include lime (the mineral complex calcium oxide, not the fruit juice) in their ingredient list. The addi-tion of lime to the cornmeal helps you absorb the niacin (vitamin B3) in the corn.
- Make a cold, nutritionally rich salad by combining cooked corn kernels, quinoa, tomatoes, green peppers, and your favorite dressing.
- Try *polenta* as a pizza crust for a gluten-free treat.

Corn comes in a variety of ways. Here is a list of the most common:

- Cornmeal is corn ground into flour. It is a staple in many parts of the world.

- Steel-ground yellow cornmeal is common in the United States. It can be kept almost indefinitely if stored in an airtight container in a cool, dry place.

- Grinding cornmeal by stone leaves some of the hull and germ, lending more flavor and nutrition to recipes. It is more perishable than steel-ground cornmeal, but will store longer if refrigerated.

def•i•ni•tion

Polenta is cornmeal made into a mush. It is versatile and can be a first course, baked, or served in place of bread.

- White cornmeal is popular in the United Sates for making cornbread.

- Blue cornmeal is made from blue corn, which is relatively rare. But beware, as food producers sometimes add blue food coloring to the cheaper and easier-to-find yellow cornmeal, so when you buy a blue corn product it may actually be made with yellow corn.

- Hominy is dried corn kernels that have been treated with mineral salts. The process dates back nearly 10,000 years to ancient Mesoamerican cultures. It converts some of the niacin (and possibly other B vitamins) into a form that our bodies can absorb more easily and it improves the availability of its amino acids. Hominy can be ground into a fine dough to make tamales and tortillas.

- Hominy grits are made from corn from which the bran and germ have been removed. They are traditional in the Southern United States.

Flax

Flax is an ancient plant; its fiber produces linen, seeds, and oil. Flax is heart-healthy because it contains alpha-linolenic acid (ALA), an important omega-3 fatty acid. Flaxseeds have a pleasant, nutty flavor and can be sprinkled on salads, cooked vegetables, or cereals. Eating too much, however, can cause an aftertaste.

Millet

Millet is highly nutritious, nonglutinous, and like buckwheat and quinoa is not an acid-forming food, so it is soothing and easy to digest. In fact, it is considered to be one of the least allergenic and most digestible grains available, and it is a warming grain so will help to heat the body in cold or rainy seasons and climates.

Millet is tasty, with a mildly sweet, nutlike flavor, and contains a myriad of beneficial nutrients. It is nearly 15 percent protein, contains high amounts of fiber, B-complex vitamins including niacin, thiamin, and riboflavin, the essential amino acid methionine, lecithin, and some vitamin E. It is particularly high in the minerals iron, magnesium, phosphorous, and potassium.

Millet's soft, cohesive texture and quick cooking make it ideal for side dishes, stuffing, burgers, and casseroles. It is great in soups, stews, and salads. The flavor of millet is enhanced by lightly roasting the grains in a dry pan before cooking. If millet is presoaked the cooking time is shortened by 5 to 10 minutes.

Oats

Oats are a reliable whole grain because they usually do not have their bran and germ removed in processing. They are gluten-free and one of the top sources of soluble fiber, which can help lower cholesterol. (Soluble fiber is able to be absorbed by the body). They have a sweet flavor that makes them a favorite for breakfast cereals.

Oats gain part of their distinctive flavor from the roasting process they undergo after being harvested and cleaned. Although oats are then hulled, this process does not strip away their bran and germ, allowing them to retain a concentrated source of their fiber and nutrients.

Oats are sold as whole grains, oat flour, oat bran, and oatmeal (rolled oats). Steel-cut oats have a pleasant nutty flavor and they do not raise blood sugar levels as high as rolled oats. However, they take longer to cook than rolled oats. Oats can be added to baked goods, to make a nondairy milklike drink, and as an ingredient in the German/Swiss breakfast cereal muesli and in granola.

Quinoa

Quinoa is another ancient grain. Botanically it is a vegetable and not a true grain. Happily, quinoa is a complete protein. In other words, it contains all the essential amino acids that our bodies can't make on their own.

Quinoa cooks in about 10 to 12 minutes, creating a light, fluffy side dish. It can be added to soups, salads, and baked goods. Quinoa cereals and other health-promoting processed foods are becoming available. Though much of our quinoa is still imported from South America, farmers in high-altitude areas near the Rockies are also beginning to cultivate quinoa.

Quinoa is a small, light-colored round grain, similar in appearance to sesame seeds. But quinoa is also available in other colors such as red (see the recipe for Big Protein Red Quinoa Salad in Chapter 3). Sometimes quinoa must be rinsed before cooking, to remove the bitter residue of saponins, a plant defense that wards off insects. So be sure to check the instructions on quinoa packaging.

Rice

Rice is an easily digested grain. It is ideal if you are on a restricted diet or are gluten-intolerant. Whole-grain rice is usually brown, but also comes in colors such as black, purple, or red. Brown rice is lower in fiber than most other whole grains. It has a mild nutty flavor, is chewier than white rice, and becomes rancid more quickly. Check for usability dates on labels, and if you buy in bulk make sure that the store has a high turnover. If stored in a tightly closed container in the refrigerator or freezer, it will stay fresh for up to a year.

If you must eat white rice, "converted rice" is parboiled before refining, a process which drives some of the B vitamins into the endosperm so that they are not lost when the bran is removed. As a result, converted rice is healthier than regular white rice, but still is lacking many nutrients found in brown rice.

Brown rice has only the outer hull removed, so it retains an impressive variety of vitamins and minerals. It is low in protein, but is relatively high in the important amino acid lysine. Because the bran is not milled away, brown rice contains four times the amount of insoluble fiber found in white rice—a prime reason for eating brown rice instead of white.

Here are some quick facts to help you distinguish between different types of rice:

◆ Long-grain brown rice stays firm when cooked.

◆ Medium-grain rice has plumper grains than those of long-grain rice. It works well in soups and stews.

◆ Short-grain sticks together when cooked and is easier to eat with chopsticks than longer-grain rices.

◆ Sweet rice, or mochi rice, is a Japanese rice that is used for desserts.

◆ Aromatic rices include texmati, basmati, and Thai jasmine rice. Aromatic rices gives off a nutty-sweet fragrance as they cook and have a sweet, delicate flavor.

◆ Quick-cooking brown rice has been precooked so that it's ready in about 10 minutes. However, it is not as nutritious as the regular variety.

Did You Know?

Here are some quick facts about rice:

◆ There are more than 7,000 varieties of rice.

◆ Asian countries produce about 90 percent of the world's rice.

◆ About one third of the rice used in the United States is found in beer.

◆ In Japan, the word for rice is the same as the word for "meal."

◆ Rice is the staple food of more than half the world's population.

Sorghum

Sorghum, also known as milo, is a gluten-free grain that is becoming popular among people who are allergic or sensitive to wheat. Although it has been part of the human diet in Africa and India for centuries, in the United States, it has been used mainly to feed livestock. This grain is also being researched for its potential as a protection against free radicals. Sorghum is high in insoluble fiber. Sorghum flour is used in baking. The nutritional value of sorghum is similar to corn. Sorghum is environmentally friendly. It is water efficient, requires little fertilizer or pesticides, and is biodegradable.

Expect to see more and more sorghum products on grocery shelves. Private industries are interested in it as a gluten-free alternative to wheat. They are busily working to improve sorghum processing for the cereal, snack food, baking, and brewing industries.

InflamWarnings

Refrigerate whole grains that you plan to have on hand for more than 2 months. During warm months, refrigerate them at all times. If you are buying in bulk make sure that you shop in a store with a high turnover of products to ensure that the grains have not been sitting around for a long time.

Spelt

Spelt is a wheat species that has been in use since Roman times. It has found a new upsurge in popularity as a health food, because it is higher in protein than common wheat. In fact, spelt production in North America has increased nearly eighty-fold in less than a decade.

Spelt retains a sturdy husk or hull that remains with the kernel, as opposed to modern wheat varieties which have been bred to lose their husks when harvested. Spelt's hull protects spelt from pollutants and insects. Spelt tends to be environmentally friendly. It is not normally treated with pesticides or other chemicals.

Spelt can be used in place of common wheat in most recipes. Spelt does contain a moderate amount of gluten, however, and is not a substitute for people with a wheat allergy or intolerance.

Triticale

Triticale is a new wonder grain that is a hybrid of durum wheat and rye. It has only been grown commercially for 35 years. Triticale looks a lot like wheat berries. It is higher in protein and lower in gluten than wheat, and has a more healthful balance of amino acids. It has double the lysine as wheat, which is an essential amino acid with many important health-promoting qualities including aiding in the growth and bone development of children.

With a slightly nutty flavor, triticale comes in several forms including whole berry, flakes, and flour. Whole triticale can be cooked and used in a variety of dishes including cereals, casseroles, and pilafs. Because triticale flour is low in gluten, bread made with it alone is quite heavy.

Wheat

Wheat contains large amounts of gluten, the stretchy protein that causes baked goods to rise. In fact, it's almost impossible to make dough rise without at least some wheat mixed in.

There are about 30 species of wheat and two main varieties. (Also see the listing for spelt above.) Durum wheat is made into pasta, while bread wheat is used for most other wheat foods.

Hard wheat has more protein, including more gluten, and is used for bread, while soft wheat creates "cake flour" with lower protein.

Whole-wheat kernels, known as wheat berries, can be cooked as a side dish or breakfast cereal, but must be boiled for about an hour, preferably after soaking overnight. Cracked wheat cooks faster.

Wheat bread and other foods made with the grain are a staple for over a third of the world's people. In fact, wheat is usually present in some form at almost every meal and in most snacks. Breads, cookies, cakes, crackers, noodles, and pasta are all made from wheat.

During the 1900s, scientists developed many new kinds of wheat. These new types of wheat can produce large amounts of grain that can resist cold, disease, insects, and other crop threats. As a result, wheat production around the world has risen dramatically.

Wild Rice

Wild rice is not technically rice at all, but the seed of an aquatic grass originally grown by indigenous tribes around the Great Lakes. Most wild rice is still harvested by Native Americans, largely in Minnesota.

The strong flavor and high price of wild rice mean that it is most often consumed in a blend with other rices or other grains. Wild rice has twice the protein and fiber of brown rice, but less iron and calcium.

Recipes

For more whole-grain recipes, see Chapter 3.

Wheat Berry Tapenade

3 cloves garlic, minced

½ tsp. Dijon mustard

1 cup pitted and finely chopped Kalamata olives

1 cup fully cooked wheat berries

1 tsp. salt

In a bowl combine all ingredients. Serve with crusty bread, on a salad, or on its own.

Fresh Corn Salsa

6 servings

1 ear fresh sweet corn

½ bunch cilantro, finely chopped

4 green onions, chopped

2 small tomatoes, diced

¼ cup lemon juice

¼ tsp. sea salt or to taste

¼ tsp. ground cumin

⅛ tsp. chili powder

Cut kernels off the cob and put them into a medium-size bowl. Add remaining ingredients and mix well. Adjust seasonings to taste, and serve chilled or at room temperature.

Kasha Pilaf

2 cups kasha

2 TB. olive oil

5 large onions, diced

2 carrots, diced

2 celery stalks, diced

3 garlic cloves, chopped

½ cup tamari

½ tsp. parsley

½ tsp. garlic powder

½ tsp. basil

¼ tsp. salt

⅛ tsp. cayenne pepper

3 TB. tahini

Simmer kasha in 4 cups water. Cook for 15 to 20 minutes, until soft. Heat oil in a skillet and add the chopped vegetables. Sauté for 7 minutes, until soft. Mix kasha and add to the vegetables.

Add tahini and seasonings and cook for 8 to 10 minutes.

Toasted Steel-Cut Oatmeal

This recipe is prepared like a pilaf.

1 cup steel-cut oats	**½ cup low-fat milk**
3 cups boiling water	**½ cup buttermilk**

Spray a large saucepot with cooking oil and add the oats. Stir for 2 minutes to toast. Add the boiling water and reduce heat to a simmer. Simmer for 25 minutes. Do not stir. Combine the milk and buttermilk and add to the oatmeal. Stir gently and cook for 10 minutes. Serve with brown sugar, berries, yogurt, or other toppings.

Gluten-Free Banana Bread

¼ cup peanuts	**¼ cup canola or other non-saturated vegetable oil**
1¾ cups amaranth flour, sifted	**¼ cup honey**
½ cup arrowroot	**2 eggs**
2 tsp. baking soda	**2 TB. lemon juice**
½ cup walnuts, chopped	**1 tsp. vanilla**
1½ cups banana, mashed	

Finely grind peanuts and mix with the flour, arrowroot, and baking soda in a large bowl. Stir in the chopped walnuts.

In a separate bowl, mix together the bananas, oil, honey, eggs, lemon juice, and vanilla. Then pour the liquid mixture into the flour bowl and gently mix with a few swift strokes.

Pour into a greased 9×5 loaf pan and bake at 350°F for 55 to 60 minutes.

The Least You Need to Know

◆ A diet rich in whole grains helps prevent inflammation and other diseases.

◆ You should eat at least three servings of whole grains per day.

◆ Whole grains are a great source of insoluble fiber.

Putting It into Action: Protein

In This Chapter

- Learn about animal and plant sources of protein
- Recognize the plethora of soy products
- Legumes: affordable wonder foods
- Recipes for an anti-inflammation diet

Along with carbohydrates and fats, protein is an important macronutrient in the human diet. Among many other things, it supplies your body with the essential amino acids that it needs.

Not getting enough protein can lead to a host of problems and can be fatal, due to the lack of material for the body to construct its own proteins. However, for most of us, the danger is not protein deficiency. It is getting too much of a good thing, along with the harmful fats that come with it.

That is why we made Principle #5: Eat healthy sources of protein. A hot dog at the ballpark is not a healthful protein. A handful or two of hot peanuts is. A barbecued steak with a pat of butter "to bring out the flavor" is not a healthful source of protein. Grilled lean chicken is. You get the picture.

In this chapter, we cover how to add healthy proteins to your diet, and which high-fat proteins you should avoid.

Protein: The Basics

There are two types of protein: complete and incomplete. *Complete proteins* contain all of the essential amino acids we need to get from our diets. Animal proteins like meat, poultry, fish, dairy products, and eggs all contain complete proteins.

def•i•ni•tion

Complete proteins contain all of the essential amino acids we need to get from our diets. Incomplete proteins don't contain all of the essential amino acids we need. As a general rule, animal proteins are complete and plant proteins are incomplete, but can be combined to make complete proteins.

Incomplete proteins don't contain all of the essential amino acids we need. With a couple of exceptions, plant proteins are incomplete.

Whether complete or incomplete, the best approach to getting enough protein in your diet is to get away from the idea of meat as the focus of every meal. If you do have meat on your menu, approach it as one part of the meal, instead of the focus. In fact, a better alternative is to make vegetables and fruits the centers of attention at mealtime. Mix things up: Include two or more vegetarian-style (meatless) meals each week. Experiment with soy and some of the protein-rich grains. And increase servings of brown rice, pasta, dry beans, and even peanuts in meals.

Animal Proteins

Lean animal proteins are healthful proteins. The best choices are fish; shellfish; skinless, lean chicken or turkey; low-fat or fat-free dairy (skim milk, low-fat cheese); egg whites; and an egg substitute.

If you are like many Americans, you love red meat. Then the best choice is to stick to lean cuts (loin and tenderloin), whether it be beef, pork, or lamb or another source. Even then, make eating red meat a rare event.

Start with a lean choice:

◆ The leanest cuts of beef are round steaks and roasts (round eye, top round, bottom round, round tip), top loin, top sirloin, and chuck shoulder and arm roasts.

◆ The leanest cuts of pork are pork loin, tenderloin, center loin, and ham.

- Choose extra-lean ground beef. The label should say at least "90% lean." You may be able to find ground beef that is 93 percent or 95 percent lean.

- Boneless, skinless chicken breasts and turkey cutlets are the leanest poultry choices.

- Choose lean turkey, roast beef, ham, or low-fat luncheon meats for sandwiches instead of luncheon meats with more fat, such as regular bologna or salami.

Keep it lean:

- Trim away all of the visible fat from meats and poultry before cooking.

- Broil, grill, roast, poach, or boil meat, poultry, or fish instead of frying.

- Drain off any fat that appears during cooking.

- Skip or limit the breading on meat, poultry, or fish. Breading adds fat and calories. It will also cause the food to soak up more fat during frying.

- Prepare dry beans and peas without added fats.

- Choose and prepare foods without high-fat sauces or gravies.

- Stay away from sausage, bacon, and other high-fat meats.

Not Just for Nickels

American buffalo is an increasingly popular option for lean protein. Also called bison, it is flavorful and tender. Surprisingly, buffalo meat provides more protein and nutrients with fewer calories and less fat than any other type of meat, including chicken. The American Heart Association includes bison in their lean-meat dietary guidelines. Buffalo can be purchased ground, bratwurst style, or as steaks or roasts. It may be used in recipes wherever beef is used.

Maybe There Is Some Truth to High-Protein Diets

Once thought to be a gimmick, high-protein diets to lose weight have gained some respect. Studies have shown that these diets may work more quickly than low-fat diets, at least in the first 6 months. After a year or so, though, weight loss is about equal. A high-protein diet that limits saturated and trans fats may reduce blood fats and be good for the heart.

One theory about why high-protein diets work is that proteins slow the movement of food from the stomach, which helps to hold off hunger pangs. In addition, protein does not cause a rise in blood sugar. And your body uses more energy to digest protein than it does to digest the other two macronutrients.

That being said, do not go overboard on protein and cut other foods from your diet or you will be deficient in important inflammation-fighting nutrients such as omega-3 fatty acids. In addition, this kind of diet effectively creates a sort-of starvation state, and can have serious health consequences.

Eggs

Eggs are rich in protein and other nutrients but are high in cholesterol, which can contribute to high blood cholesterol levels, a major risk factor for heart disease and stroke. In fact, one egg contains about 213 milligrams of cholesterol, about 71 percent of the daily recommended limit. However, the culprit is the egg yolk. Egg whites have no cholesterol. Limit the amount of whole eggs you eat and substitute with other sources of protein. When baking use two egg whites, or one egg white plus 2 teaspoons of unsaturated oil, in place of one whole egg.

Milk Products

Although milk products are high in protein, they are also high in saturated fat. Choose from the following sources and stay away from whole milk, butter, ice cream, and other high-fat dairy products:

- Skim, fat-free, zero-fat, no-fat, or nonfat milk
- ½ percent low-fat milk
- 1 percent low-fat milk
- Nonfat or low-fat dry milk powder
- Evaporated skim or fat-free milk
- Buttermilk made from fat-free or 1 percent fat milk
- Nonfat or low-fat yogurt (and frozen)
- Nonfat or low-fat cheeses
- Nonfat or low-fat ice cream

Plants and Protein

Plant foods contain the same eight amino acids that animal proteins have, but in different amounts. But they do not carry significant amounts of fat with them, so they are a great staple for the anti-inflammation diet.

As long as you are eating a healthy diet, plant foods can supply you all of the amino acids you need. The often-quoted phrase at weddings, "the power of two," applies to plant proteins. When you put two incomplete proteins together, the result is a complete protein. Examples of incomplete proteins that become complete proteins when combined are: rice and beans, corn and beans, and milk and cereal.

Dr. Walter Willett, the developer of the Healthy Eating Pyramid, which provided the background for our seven principles, states, "In terms of your health, there isn't enough evidence to argue that one type of protein is better for you than another." Dr. Willett says animal and vegetable proteins have roughly equivalent effects on health.

Good news: the idea that two incomplete proteins have to be eaten at the same meal to create a complete protein is a myth. Studies show that incomplete proteins can be eaten as much as 24 hours a part. Your body will effectively combine all the amino acids you eat during that time period. So, if you eat a balanced diet (remember Principle #1?), you don't need to worry too much about whether your proteins are "complete" or "incomplete" proteins.

And here is more good news: all plant proteins are more economical sources of protein than animal products, and because they are farther down on the food chain, they are friendlier to the environment.

Soy Proteins

For such a little bean, they pack a protein wallop. Soy foods contain high-quality protein. Their protein content is roughly equal to the quality of animal proteins. However, soy is not without its critics in terms of health benefits and digestibility. More about that later in Chapter 10.

New soy products are appearing on grocery shelves every day, in large part because the U.S. Food and Drug Administration (FDA) authorized a nutrition label to be put on soy foods claiming that at least 25 grams of soy protein a day, as part of a low-fat diet, can lower blood cholesterol levels in people who have high cholesterol. Soy products containing at least 6.25 grams of soy protein per serving are allowed to bear the FDA-approved health claim label.

Soybean products range from liquid to solid, smooth to lumpy, and tasty to yucky (the latter depending on your taste buds and point of view). They include soy flour, soy sauce, texturized vegetable protein (TVP), soy cheese, soy milk, tempeh, tofu, soy sauce, soy cheese, soy flakes, soy grits, soy nuts, and meat alternatives.

The following describe these products:

◆ Soy flour is made by grinding roasted soybeans into a fine powder. It contains almost three times the amount of protein as wheat flour. It may be used in a number of ways, including adding it to sauces and gravies as a thickener, or to pancake batter for a nutty flavor and protein boost. Soy flour does not have gluten so it cannot completely replace wheat flour in a dough that requires yeast.

◆ Soy sauce is a staple of Chinese food and cooking. It is derived from fermented soybeans mixed with roasted grain (wheat, barley, or rice are common), injected with a special yeast mold, and flavored with salt. Varieties include light, dark, mushroom soy sauce, and tamari. Even though soy sauce is derived from soy, it is actually a weak source of protein. A fourth of a cup of soy sauce has only 1 gram of protein.

If you are sensitive to gluten or yeast be sure to read the labels on all soy-type sauces.

InflamWarnings

Even reduced-sodium soy sauce is relatively high in sodium. Use it in small amounts if you are salt sensitive. Be careful of soy sauce labeled as "light." It is actually saltier than the darker varieties, and should not be confused with low-sodium, reduced-sodium, or "lite" soy sauces.

Here are some facts about soy products:

◆ Texturized vegetable protein (TVP) is protein that has been taken from soybeans. Low in fat and rich in protein, TVP adds flavor and texture to foods. However, it often takes some getting used to when used in sauces, casseroles, stews, and other entrées. TVP is available to consumers in powder form, chunks, slices, and granules.

◆ Soy cheese is a cheese substitute made from soy milk. However, using the word "cheese" to describe these products is really unfair. Soft soy cheese is used in place of sour cream or cream cheese. Firmer cheeses do not melt the way dairy cheeses do, but are usually billed as dairy cheese replacements.

Caution: firmer soy cheese is often colored and/or flavored to imitate specific dairy cheeses, such as mozzarella or cheddar. In addition, if you are sensitive to milk products, check the label of soy cheeses carefully, as they may contain dairy proteins such as whey or casein.

◆ Soy grits are toasted, cracked soybeans that are usually the size of very coarse cornmeal. Soy flakes are cracked soybeans that have been pressed through rollers (like rolled oats). Grits are high in protein and may be cooked like rice and used in pilafs. Soy flakes are cooked like rolled oats and served as a hot cereal.

◆ Miso is a fermented soybean paste used for seasoning and in soup stock. Higher in protein than soy sauce, 1 ounce has 3 grams of protein.

◆ Meat alternatives imitate hot dogs, bacon, and other meats.

◆ Soy protein isolate is a dry powder food ingredient that is made from defatted soy meal. It has been separated or isolated from the other components of the soybean, making it 90 to 95 percent pure protein and nearly carbohydrate- and fat-free with a very mild flavor. Soy protein isolate can be purchased as flavored soy protein shake powder or plain soy isolate powder. Several brands are fortified with calcium and other minerals and vitamins, along with sweeteners and flavorings. Individual, single-serve packages are the utmost in convenience for busy consumers. The most economical form of soy isolate is plain powder, with no other ingredients added.

Soy protein isolate is sold in the health-food section or the pharmacy within the regular supermarket. Natural food supermarkets and health-food stores carry the widest variety of products. Other sources for soy protein isolate powders are mail order, food cooperatives, buying clubs, on-line shopping, and mass-market stores. Soy protein isolate is used in making a variety of foods. It may be found in …

◆ Dairy-type products such as beverage powders, infant formulas, and liquid nutritional meals.

◆ Bottled fruit drinks.

◆ Power bars.

◆ Soups and sauces.

◆ Meat analogs that resemble conventional foods in color, texture, and taste.

◆ Breads and baked goods.

◆ Breakfast cereals.

◆ Tempeh is a solid made by the controlled fermentation of cooked soybeans. It has been a favorite food and major source of protein in Indonesia for hundreds of years, and is gaining in popularity here. Tempeh has a firm texture and a mushroom flavor. It can replace mushrooms in recipes. Often it is sliced and fried.

◆ Tofu, also known as soybean curd, is a soft food made by curdling fresh hot soy milk with a coagulant such as nigari, a compound found in natural ocean water, or calcium sulfate, a naturally occurring mineral. Curds also can be produced by acidic foods like lemon juice or vinegar. The curds then are generally pressed into a solid block.

Tofu is a dietary staple throughout Asia. It is made daily in thousands of tofu shops and sold on the street. Tofu soaks up any flavor that is added to it.

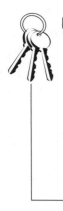

InflamWise

Three main types of tofu are available in grocery stores:

◆ Firm tofu is dense and solid. It has a higher concentration of protein than other forms of tofu.

◆ Soft tofu is much less dense. It is great for blending into dressings and sauces. It can be used to reduce the amount of egg used in a recipe and to replace sour cream or yogurt. Soft tofu also is lower in protein than firm tofu.

◆ Silken tofu is made by a slightly different process that results in a creamy, custardlike product. Silken tofu also is available in extra firm, firm, and soft.

◆ Soy nuts are made from whole soybeans that have been soaked in water and then baked. They are a great high-protein snack food similar in texture and flavor to peanuts. Soy nuts can be found in different flavors, such as chili or paprika.

Soy's Tainted Reputation

Because the FDA allowed soy producers to make a health claim about their products, soy has been the center of controversy. The plethora of information out there for and against soy can be confusing. Here is our bottom line: soy foods are good for fighting inflammation when they replace less healthful choices, like red meat.

But keep this in mind: soy by itself is not a magic bullet. Commenting on the heart-benefit claims for soy, Dr. Willett put it this way: "It will work only if it is part of an otherwise healthy diet." Dr. Willett and his colleagues suggest keeping your servings of soy to two or four times a week. Dr. Willett is cautious about soy products because of their phytoestrogens, which are "potent biological agents" similar to the hormone estrogen. Until we know more about phytoestrogens, he does not feel that we should be eating a lot of soy every day.

How Much Protein Is in Soy?

Just how much protein is in soy? Here are some guidelines:

- Four ounces of firm tofu contains 13 grams of soy protein.
- One soy "sausage" link provides 6 grams of protein.
- One soy "burger" includes 10 to 12 grams of protein.
- An 8-ounce glass of plain soy milk contains 10 grams of protein.
- One soy protein bar has 14 grams of protein.
- One half cup of tempeh provides 19.5 grams of protein.
- One quarter cup of roasted soy nuts contains 19 grams of soy protein.

The Taste of Soy

If you are not already eating soy products, it may take some time getting used to the taste. The American Dietetic Association recommends introducing soy slowly by adding small amounts to your daily diet or mixing into existing foods. Then, after the taste and texture have become familiar, add more.

Also try the following further suggestions for adding soy to the diet:

- Include soy-based beverages, muffins, sausages, yogurt, or cream cheese at breakfast.
- Use soy deli meats, soy nut butter (similar to peanut butter), or soy cheese to make sandwiches.
- Top pizzas with soy cheese, pepperoni, sausages, or soy crumbles (similar to ground beef).
- Grill soy hot dogs, burgers, marinated tempeh, or baked tofu.
- Cube and stir-fry tofu or tempeh and add to a salad.
- Pour soy milk on cereal and use it in cooking or to make "smoothies."

◆ Order soy-based dishes such as spicy bean curd and miso soup at Asian restaurants.

◆ Try roasted soy nuts or a soy protein bar for a snack.

Eating Soy Can be Embarrassing

Soy products can cause stomach problems including flatus (gas), bloating, and rumbling intestines due to indigestible carbohydrates. Soy products that are more processed are less likely to be a problem. For example, soy isolate tends to be less gas-forming because many of the indigestible carbohydrates have been removed. A product called Beano helps many people. It works with your body's digestion to break down gassy foods, making them more digestible.

Legumes: Affordable Wonder Foods

Also known as pulses, there are over 1,000 species of legumes. Legumes have been found in 5,000-year-old settlements across the globe from the Eastern Mediterranean to Switzerland. They are the edible seeds of plants.

Legumes are truly wonder foods because they are low in fat, high in protein, and absorb the flavor of spices and herbs. Beans and other legumes have many nutrients now recognized as important in preventing heart disease, cancer, and obesity. They are also high in complex carbohydrates, fiber, vitamins, and minerals. And they are easy on the budget, hence their nickname, "the poor man's meat."

Legumes are eaten with the skin still intact, split in half, or without their skins. If you are a vegetarian, lentils are probably a staple in your diet. If you are a meat eater, legumes offer an alternative source of protein without the fat but with a lot of fiber.

Lentils are 20 to 25 percent protein, double that found in wheat and three times that found in rice. However, they are poor in the essential amino acid methionine. When eaten with grains they are a complete protein.

There are many classes of dry beans produced in the United States. The major ones are adzuki, anasazi, black, blackeye, chickpea (large or small), cranberry, Great Northern, kidney (dark red, light red, or white/cannellini), lima (baby or large), marrow (white), navy (pea), pink, red (small), pinto, white (small), and yellow eye.

Beans Can Be Embarrassing, Too

Like soybeans, beans are known to cause stomach discomfort. If they are soaked in water for at least a few hours (preferably overnight), they are much easier to cook and cause less flatulence.

Nuts to That

Nuts are often looked over as the elegant source of protein that they are. Yes, nuts are high in fat, but the fat is heart-healthy, and may help lower low-density lipoproteins. In fact, nuts are recommended as part of the DASH diet (Dietary Approaches to Stop Hypertension), a dietary plan clinically proven to significantly reduce blood pressure. The DASH diet is supported by the National Heart, Lung, and Blood Institute and recommends four to five servings per week of "nuts, seeds, and legumes."

The Food and Drug Administration recommends eating up to 1.5 ounces of nuts daily. Here are some tips:

◆ A handful of nuts equals about 1 ounce.

◆ On average, a 1.5-ounce serving is equivalent to about ⅓ cup of nuts.

◆ In terms of protein, ⅓ cup of nuts or 2 tablespoons of peanut butter equals about 1 ounce of meat.

The following table gives the approximate number of nuts per ounce and an overview of calories, protein, and fat.

Nutrients in 1 Ounce (28 Grams) of Shelled Tree Nuts and Peanuts

Nut(s)	Amt./oz.	Calories	Protein	Total Fat	Sat	Mono	Poly
Almonds	20–24	160	6g	14g	1g	9g	3g
Brazil	6–8	190	4	19	5	7	7
Cashews	16–18	160	4	13	3	8	2
Hazelnuts	18–20	180	4	17	2	13	2
Macadamias	10–12	200	2	22	3	17	0.5
Peanuts	28	170	7	14	2	7	4
Pecan halves	18–20	200	3	20	2	12	6
Pine Nuts	150–157	160	7	14	2	5	6
Pistachios	45–47	160	6	13	1.5	7	4
Walnut halves	14	190	4	18	1.5	2.5	13

Source: University of Nebraska Cooperative Extension.

Try These Grains for Protein Variety

The grains amaranth and quinoa have the distinction of being complete proteins. We covered details about them in Chapter 8. Try them out as protein sources to provide variety to your diet.

Recipes

Soy Nuts

Soy nuts are easy to make. Soak dry soy beans in enough water to cover for 3 hours. Then drain and spread the soy nuts in one layer on a well-oiled cookie sheet. Roast at 350°F, stirring often, until well browned. Add salt and desired spices to taste. Store in an airtight container.

Blender Peanut Butter

Makes 1 cup creamy or 1½ cups crunchy peanut butter

2 cups roasted shelled peanuts	**½ tsp. (only if using unsalted peanuts)**
3 tsp. peanut oil	**For crunchy: ½ cup chopped roasted peanuts**

Place ingredients in blender. With the lid secured, blend until mixture becomes pastelike or spreadable (3 to 4 minutes). For crunchy peanut butter, stir in additional nuts after the blending is completed.

Store in a tightly closed container in the refrigerator. Oil may rise to the top. If this occurs, stir before using.

≈‿

Buffalo Stew

2 lb. buffalo meat, cubed	1 tsp. oregano
¼ cup olive oil	1 tsp. salt
2 large chopped onions	½ tsp. pepper
2 cloves of minced garlic	4 carrots, sliced
8 cups fat-free beef broth	1 potato, cubed
2 cups corn	1 green pepper, chopped

Brown buffalo in oil. Put meat aside and sauté garlic and onions in the oil. Return meat to pan, add broth, corn, oregano, salt, and pepper. Cook for 2 hours, or until meat is tender. Add carrots, potato, and green pepper and continue to cook until done, about 30 minutes.

The Least You Need to Know

- Eating a well-balanced variety of wholesome foods will ensure that you get all of the amino acids you need.

- Pay attention to the fats that come along with the proteins you eat.

- Eat only lean meats.

- Eat soy as a source of protein, but only in moderation.

- Try other options for getting protein, such as quinoa, amaranth, buffalo, legumes, or nuts.

Chapter 10

Putting It into Action: Fruits and Vegetables

In This Chapter

◆ Discover how fruits and vegetables fight inflammation

◆ Learn about the phytochemicals and vitamins in fruits and vegetables, and their role in the anti-inflammation diet

◆ Understand the guidelines for fitting produce into your diet

◆ Learn some tips for grilling fruits and vegetables

Fruits and vegetables should be key parts of your daily diet. Often called "produce" by grocers, eating plenty of different kinds of fruits and vegetables can help prevent inflammation and protect you against many chronic diseases. They are also great for your digestive system.

Most of us eat fewer servings of produce than we should. To help prevent inflammation and foster health, you should eat at least five servings a day. But we would actually like you to aim much higher—five a day should be a minimum.

This chapter covers important information about Principle #6, "eating plenty of fruits and vegetables," and provides tips on how to fit them into your diet.

Fruits and Vegetables Fight Inflammation

We've always known that eating fruits and vegetables is good for us, but no one had examined their anti-inflammatory characteristics until recently. Now the first study to look at the link gives us some evidence. The research, reported in the *American Journal of Clinical Nutrition*, suggests that eating lots of fruits and vegetables reduces C-reactive protein levels, which means that it reduces levels of inflammation.

Researchers recruited 3,258 men between ages 60 to 69 with no history of diabetes or heart disease to eat a low-produce diet for a month and then indulge in eight servings a day. When the men changed from a diet low in fruits and vegetables to one high in them, they experienced a significant drop in CRP.

Another study has shown that the fiber in fruits and vegetables, along with that found in legumes and grains (see Chapters 8 and 9) can help ease inflammation. The study included 524 healthy women and men. The results of this study also appeared in the *American Journal of Clinical Nutrition*.

The study's participants, who were mostly overweight or obese, had their CRP levels measured and their diets analyzed every three months over one year. Those who ate the most fiber had 63 percent lower CRP concentrations than those who ate the least.

The study also found that both soluble and insoluble fibers from diets were linked with lower CRP levels. (See Chapter 8 for a description of the two types of fiber.)

Scientists are looking into these issues further. But for now, make sure that your diet includes lots of fruits and vegetables.

Produce and Disease

Fruits and vegetables are good for your heart, brain, eyes, and general good health. Here are some facts about their benefits:

- As mentioned in Chapter 4, a study conducted at Harvard showed that those who averaged eight or more servings of produce a day were 30 percent less likely to have a heart attack or stroke than those who ate less than one-and-a-half servings a day.

- Results of the Dietary Approaches to Stop Hypertension (DASH) study found that people with high blood pressure who followed the diet—which is high in produce and low-fat dairy products and low in saturated and total fat—reduced their systolic blood pressure as much as medications did.

◆ In the National Heart, Lung, and Blood Institute's Family Heart Study, men and women who ate more than four servings of produce a day had significantly lower levels of LDL (bad) cholesterol than those with lower consumption.

◆ Researchers in Italy found that a daily glass of tomato juice could lower inflammation by over 30 percent after 6 weeks of supplementing a normal diet with the juice. Research also suggests that tomatoes may help protect men against aggressive forms of prostate cancer. One of the pigments that give tomatoes their red hue—lycopene—could be involved in this protective effect. However, more research is needed to confirm this connection.

◆ A study of 68,535 women from the Instituto Nacional de Salud Publica in Mexico reported that women who ate a diet high in fruits and vegetables (such as tomatoes, carrots, and leafy vegetables) considerably reduced their risk of asthma. After 11 years of follow-up, the researchers found that women who consumed more than 90 grams per day of leafy vegetables had a 22 percent lower risk of asthma than those who ate less than 40 grams per day. Similar risk reductions were also seen for tomatoes (20 percent) and carrots (18 percent).

◆ Several recent studies have shown a strong link between nutrition and the development of macular degeneration. People with diets high in fruits and vegetables (especially leafy green vegetables) have a lower incidence of macular degeneration. More studies are needed to determine if nutritional supplements can prevent progression in patients with existing disease.

Produce and Weight

Fruits and vegetables are mainstays of diets. Because they're low in calories and high in fiber, fruits and vegetables can help you control your weight. By eating more produce and fewer high-calorie foods, you'll find it much easier to control your weight.

Produce and Energy

Busy lives require food that's nutritious, energizing, and easy to eat on the go, like fresh fruits and vegetables. Fruits and vegetables are a natural source of energy and give the body many nutrients you need to keep going. Get your sugar fixes from produce rather than processed and refined sources.

Fruits and Vegetables 101

Produce has more going on than meets the eye. For example, tomatoes, avocados, and squashes all look like vegetables, but are actually fruits.

All fruits and vegetables are rich in nutrients. Technically, fruits are plants that contain seeds. They tend to taste sweet. Vegetables come from the rest of the plant.

Produce varies greatly in its nutrient content. For example, some are excellent sources of vitamin C, which is necessary for the growth and repair of body tissues. Others are great sources of folate, which helps produce and maintain new cells, and is particularly beneficial for pregnant women and their babies. Still others supply lots of potassium, which is important for muscles to function well and for maintaining the health of body cells.

def•i•ni•tion

Phytochemicals are sometimes called **phytonutrients**. They are substances found in plants that are not required for normal functioning of the body. However, they can have a positive effect on health and possibly eliminate disease.

All produce has fiber. Most are naturally low in fat and calories and are filling. Dark-green leafy vegetables, deeply colored fruits, and dry beans and peas are especially rich in many nutrients.

Fruits and vegetables also have health-promoting *phytochemicals*, which have been dubbed "superfoods." Phytochemicals are substances in plants that are thought to be remarkable health boosters.

Over 1,000 phytochemicals have been identified, and each fruit and vegetable has its own special array of them. However, the truth is that we just don't know enough about the action of phytochemicals to say we know for sure that they will have certain effects.

A couple phytochemicals are particularly interesting for their possible inflammation-fighting properties:

- The phrase "an apple a day keeps the doctor away" may come from the phytochemical quercetin, which is found in apples as well as onions and black tea. It is a type of flavonoid that is thought to be an anti-inflammatory. (Flavonoids are substances that give plants their colors.)

  Quercetin may help people with asthma by reducing inflammation in the airways and preventing the release of histamine (which causes congestion). It also appears to block allergic reactions to pollen, and it may help control Crohn's disease, macular degeneration, and gout.

◆ Carotenoids are phytochemicals that are the pigments responsible for the colors of many red, green, yellow, and orange fruits and vegetables. They can be converted to vitamin A. The carotenoids family includes alpha-carotene, beta-carotene, lutein, lycopene, cryptoxanthin, canthaxanthin, and zeaxanthin.

Some studies suggest that diets rich in carotenoids decrease inflammation. A small Swedish study of rheumatoid arthritis sufferers who ate a Mediterranean diet (including lots of vegetables and fruits) for 3 months found that it reduced inflammation and enhanced joint function.

InflamWise _____

Here is a reminder about the Mediterranean diet, which we talk about in Chapter 1:

The traditional foods of the Mediterranean region come from a diversity of sun-drenched plants. People in the region traditionally eat lots of fruits, vegetables, whole grains, beans, nuts, and seeds. Olive oil is the area's principle source of fat, and fish and meats are served only on special occasions.

Carotenoids may also protect your body by decreasing the risk of heart disease, stroke, blindness, and certain types of cancer. They may also help slow the aging process. Fruits and vegetables that are dark green, yellow, orange, or red contain carotenoids.

Other phytochemicals in fruits and vegetables that research has suggested may be health-promoting include the following:

◆ Beta-carotene is an *antioxidant* and may curb the damage that free radicals can do to the body. Beta-carotene also may help to slow the aging process, reduce the risk of certain types of cancer, improve lung function, and reduce complications associated with diabetes. It can be found in yellow, orange, and green leafy fruits and vegetables including carrots, spinach, lettuce, tomatoes, sweet potatoes, broccoli, cantaloupe, orange, and winter squash. As a rule of thumb, the greater the intensity of the color of the fruit or vegetable, the more beta-carotene it contains.

InflamWise _____

You may hear experts promoting the elimination of nightshade vegetables to cure arthritis. (Nightshade vegetables are tomatoes, potatoes, peppers, and eggplants.) There is no scientific information to support this claim.

◆ Lutein has been shown to reduce the risk of cataracts and macular degeneration, the leading causes of blindness in older people, and may help reduce the risk of certain types of cancer. Kale, spinach, and collard greens contain the most lutein of any fruit or vegetable. Other sources of lutein include kiwifruit, broccoli, collard greens, Brussels sprouts, Swiss chard, and romaine lettuce.

◆ Lycopene-rich diets have been shown to reduce the risk of prostate cancer and heart disease. Lycopene is found in red fruits and vegetables such as tomatoes and cooked tomato products, red peppers, pink grapefruit, and watermelon.

◆ Zeaxanthin may help to prevent macular degeneration, which is the leading cause of blindness in older people. It may also help to prevent certain types of cancer. Corn, spinach, winter squash, and egg yolks contain zeaxanthin.

◆ Flavonoids are another large family of protective phytochemicals found in fruits and vegetables. Flavonoids, also called bioflavonoids, act as antioxidants.

def•i•ni•tion

Antioxidants reduce or stop highly destructive molecules, called *free radicals,* from attacking the cells of our bodies. Free radical damage is believed to contribute to health problems such as cancer, heart disease, and aging, due to a variety of circumstances such as exposure to radiation and environment chemicals.

There are many different types of flavonoids, and each appears to have protective health effects. Some of the better known are resveratrol, anthocyanins, hesperidin, tangeritin, phenolic compounds, ellagic acid, sulphoraphane, indoles, and allium. Flavonoids are found in a variety of foods, such as oranges, kiwifruit, grapefruit, tangerines, berries, apples, red grapes, red wine, broccoli, onions, and green tea. The following explains the role of each flavonoid:

◆ Resveratrol may reduce the risk of heart disease, cancer, blood clots, and stroke. Red grapes, red grape juice, and red wine contain resveratrol.

◆ Anthocyanins, which are particularly high in blueberries, have been shown to protect against the signs of aging. In one study, elderly rats that ate the equivalent of a half cup of blueberries daily for 8 weeks improved balance, coordination, and short-term memory. Scientists think these results may apply to humans as well.

Anthocyanins in blueberries and cranberries have also been shown to help prevent urinary tract infections. Cherries, strawberries, kiwifruit, and plums also contain anthocyanins.

◆ Hesperidin may protect against heart disease. It is found in citrus fruits and fruit juices, such as oranges and orange juice, grapefruit and grapefruit juice, tangerines, lemons, limes, mandarins, and tangelos.

◆ Tangeritin may help prevent cancers of the head and neck. Animal research suggests it may be a cholesterol-lowering agent and protect against Parkinson's disease. It is found in grapefruit, oranges, and other citrus fruits and their juices.

◆ Phenolic compounds may reduce the risk of heart disease and certain types of cancer. They are found in berries, prunes, red grapes and red grape juice, kiwifruit, currants, apples and apple juice, and tomatoes.

◆ Ellagic acid may reduce the risk of certain types of cancer and decrease cholesterol levels. It is found in red grapes, kiwifruit, blueberries, raspberries, strawberries, blackberries, and currants.

◆ Sulphoraphane may reduce the risk of colon cancer. It is found in cruciferous vegetables such as broccoli sprouts, broccoli, cauliflower, kale, Brussels sprouts, cabbage, bok choy, collard greens, and turnips and turnip greens. Johns Hopkins scientists discovered that broccoli sprouts are particularly rich in sulphoraphane.

◆ Indoles may reduce the risk of certain types of cancer. Indoles are found in cruciferous vegetables, such as broccoli, cauliflower, kale, Brussels sprouts, cabbage, bok choy, collard greens, watercress, and turnips and turnip greens.

◆ Allium compounds are known for their presence in garlic, which is one of the most widely studied medicinal plants. They are being studied for several uses, including their potential benefit in reducing heart disease risk. Besides garlic, allium is also found in onions, chives, leeks, and scallions.

What Color Is Your Produce?

A good way to get a rich variety of produce in your diet is to think in terms of color. The USDA calls this "sampling the spectrum." Here are some guidelines:

◆ Reds: Lycopene and anthocyanins.

◆ Greens: Indoles, lutein, and zeaxanthin.

◆ Oranges/Yellows: Beta-carotene and bioflavonoids. Also rich in vitamin C.

◆ Blues/Purples: Flavonoids, anthocyanins, phenolics, and other phytochemicals. Blueberries, in particular, are rich in vitamin C and folic acid and high in fiber and potassium.

◆ Whites: Allicin, indoles, and sulfaforaphanes.

Savor the spectrum all year long by putting something of every color on your plate or in your lunch bag, and you are more likely to eat the recommended five to nine servings of vegetables and fruits every day. Think color: 1 cup of dark, leafy salad greens with white onions sprinkled on top, ½ cup of red tomatoes, ½ cup of yellow pineapple chunks, 6 ounces of orange juice, and ½ cup of blueberries.

How Many a Day?

How many fruits and vegetables should you eat every day? Variety should be the rule when it comes to fruits and vegetables. No single fruit or vegetable provides all of the nutrients you need. The key lies in the mixture of different fruits and vegetables that you eat.

The latest guideline from the U.S. Department of Agriculture is four servings (four ½ cups) of fruits a day and five servings (five ½ cups) of vegetables for a person who eats a 2,000-calorie diet. Specifically, they recommend the following for vegetables:

◆ Dark-green vegetables: 3 cups/week

◆ Orange vegetables: 2 cups/week

◆ Legumes (dry beans): 3 cups/week

◆ Starchy vegetables: 3 cups/week

◆ Other vegetables: 6½ cups/week

But we think it is unrealistic to think anyone can keep track of this for any length of time, so we suggest sticking with nine daily servings and thinking variety.

That being said, the amount of fruit you need to eat depends on age, sex, and level of physical activity. For more information about this, see Chapter 12. However, follow this rule: the more, the better. And the more variety, the better yet.

Supplements or Pills Are Not the Answer

Fruits and vegetables contain thousands of phytochemicals that promote health and prevent disease. When you eat produce, the phytochemicals are easily absorbed to provide the maximum health benefits. In contrast, supplements or pills that contain large doses of only one or two phytochemicals have not proven to be effective or even safe. For example, Dr. Cannon emphasizes that vitamin B6 and vitamin E supplements have been found NOT to benefit the heart as previously thought.

Is Chocolate a Fruit?

Surprise! One of the plant foods that is a superfood is dark chocolate. It is loaded with health-promoting antioxidants that may help lower blood pressure and promote vascular health. But to make the grade as a super food, the chocolate must contain at least 70 percent cocoa solids.

Hershey's produces an extra dark chocolate that touts antioxidant power equal to three cups of tea, two glasses of red wine, or 1⅓ cups of blueberries. And Dove Dark, made by Mars, Inc., contains a cocoa that contains superhigh levels of antioxidants.

InflamWise

To help protect yourself and your family from pesticides on fruits and vegetables, remove the outer leaves of leafy vegetables and then rinse the vegetables. Peel hard-skinned produce, or rinse it with lots of warm water mixed with salt and lemon juice or vinegar. Alternatively, you may want to buy and serve organic produce. Organic growers do not use pesticides to produce their fruits and vegetables.

Calculating Portions: Fruits

Principle #6 says to eat plenty of fruits and vegetables. But what does "plenty" mean? It's a good bet that it is a lot more than you eat now. The average American gets a total of just three servings of fruits and vegetables a day.

A serving of fruits and vegetables is a lot smaller than most people think. A quick guideline is that it should fit within the palm of your hand, but more specific guidelines follow.

Commonly Eaten Fruits

Some commonly eaten fruits include the following:

- Apples
- Apricots
- Avocadoes
- Bananas
- Berries such as strawberries, blueberries, raspberries, and cherries
- Grapefruit
- Grapes
- Kiwifruit
- Lemons
- Limes
- Mangoes
- Melons such as cantaloupe, honeydew, watermelon, and nectarines
- Oranges
- Peaches
- Pears
- Papayas
- Pineapple
- Plums
- Prunes
- Raisins
- Tangerines
- 100 percent fruit juice: orange, apple, grape, and grapefruit

Fruit Servings

According to the U.S. Department of Agriculture, a serving of fruit is equal to a half cup. The following specific amounts count as 1 cup of fruit—or two servings:

- Apple: half large (3.25-inch diameter); one small (2.5-inch diameter); 1 cup sliced or chopped, raw or cooked
- Applesauce: 1 cup
- Banana: 1 cup sliced, 1 large (8 to 9 inches long)
- Cantaloupe: 1 cup diced or melon balls
- Grapefruit: one medium (4-inch diameter), 1 cup sections
- Grapes: 1 cup whole or cut up, 32 seedless grapes
- Orange: one large (3¹⁄₁₆-inch diameter), 1 cup sections

◆ Peach: one large (2¾-inch diameter); 1 cup sliced or diced, raw, cooked, or canned, drained; two halves, canned

◆ Pear: one medium pear (2½ per pound); 1 cup sliced or diced, raw, cooked, or canned, drained

◆ Pineapple: 1 cup chunks, sliced, or crushed, raw, cooked or canned, drained

◆ Strawberries: About eight large berries; 1 cup whole, halved, or sliced, fresh or frozen

◆ Watermelon: one small wedge (1 inch thick); 1 cup diced or balls

◆ Dried fruits: ½ cup

Figuring Out Servings: Vegetables

Any vegetable or 100 percent vegetable juice counts as a member of the vegetable group. Vegetables may be raw or cooked, fresh, frozen, canned, or dried/dehydrated. There are five main types of vegetables: dark-green vegetables, orange vegetables, dry beans and peas, starchy vegetables, and other vegetables.

Vegetable choices should be selected from among the vegetable subgroups. It is not necessary to eat vegetables from each subgroup daily. However, over a week, try to consume the amounts listed from each subgroup as a way to reach your daily intake recommendation.

One serving (½ cup) of vegetables can include the following:

◆ 1 cup of raw leafy vegetables

◆ ½ cup of other vegetables, cooked or raw

◆ ¾ cup of vegetable juice

What counts as a cup of vegetables? In general, 1 cup of raw or cooked vegetables or vegetable juice, or 2 cups of raw leafy greens can be considered as 1 cup from the vegetable group. The list below provides the amounts that count as a cup of vegetables.

The following lists important types of dark-green vegetables.

Dark-Green Vegetables

◆ Broccoli: 1 cup chopped or florets; three spears 5 inches long, raw or cooked

◆ Greens (collards, mustard greens, turnip greens, kale): 1 cup cooked

◆ Spinach: 1 cup cooked; 2 cups raw is equivalent to 1 cup of vegetables

◆ Raw leafy greens (spinach, romaine, watercress, dark-green leafy lettuce, endive, escarole): 2 cups raw is equivalent to 1 cup of vegetables

Orange vegetables include these:

◆ Carrots: 1 cup strips, slices, or chopped, raw or cooked; two medium whole; 1 cup baby carrots (about 12)

◆ Pumpkin: 1 cup mashed, cooked

◆ Sweet potato: one large baked (2¼ inch or more diameter); 1 cup sliced or mashed, cooked

◆ Winter squash (acorn, butternut, hubbard): 1 cup cubed, cooked

Dry beans and peas (also see Chapter 9) include the following:

◆ Dry beans and peas (such as black, garbanzo, kidney, pinto, or soy beans, or black-eyed peas or split peas): 1 cup whole or mashed, cooked

◆ Tofu: 1 cup ½-inch cubes (about 8 ounces)

Starchy vegetables include these:

◆ Corn, yellow or white: 1 cup; one large ear (8 to 9 inches long)

◆ Green peas: 1 cup

Other vegetables include the following:

◆ Bean sprouts: 1 cup cooked

◆ Cabbage, green: 1 cup, chopped or shredded raw, or cooked

◆ Cauliflower: 1 cup pieces or florets, raw or cooked

◆ Celery: 1 cup, diced or sliced, raw or cooked; two large stalks (11 to 12 inches long)

- Cucumbers: 1 cup raw, sliced or chopped

- Green or wax bean: 1 cup cooked

- Green or red peppers: 1 cup chopped, raw or cooked; one large pepper (3 inches diameter, 3¾ inches long)

- Lettuce, iceberg or head: 2 cups raw, shredded or chopped

- Mushrooms: 1 cup raw or cooked

- Onions: 1 cup chopped, raw or cooked

- Tomatoes: one large raw whole (3 inches); 1 cup chopped or sliced, raw, canned, or cooked

- Tomato or mixed vegetable juice: 1 cup

- Summer squash or zucchini: 1 cup cooked, sliced or diced

Nutrients

Fruits and vegetables are chock-full of nutrition. Here are some facts about them:

Most fruits and vegetables are naturally low in fat, sodium, and calories. None have cholesterol.

Fruits and vegetables are important sources of many nutrients, including potassium, dietary fiber, vitamin C, and folate (folic acid).

Diets rich in potassium may help to maintain healthy blood pressure. Fruit sources of potassium include bananas, prunes and prune juice, dried peaches and apricots, cantaloupe, honeydew melon, and orange juice.

Dietary fiber from fruits and vegetables, as part of an overall healthy diet, helps reduce blood cholesterol levels and may lower risk of heart disease. Fiber is important for proper bowel function. It helps reduce constipation and diverticulosis.

Fiber-containing foods help provide a feeling of fullness with fewer calories. Whole or cut-up fruits are sources of dietary fiber; fruit juices contain little or no fiber.

Vitamin C is important for growth and repair of all body tissues, helps heal cuts and wounds, and keeps teeth and gums healthy.

Folate (folic acid) helps the body form red blood cells. Women of childbearing age who may become pregnant and those in the first trimester of pregnancy should consume adequate folate, including folic acid from fortified foods or supplements. This reduces the risk of developmental problems in the baby.

Vitamin A keeps eyes and skin healthy and helps to protect against infections.

Vitamin E helps protect vitamin A and essential fatty acids from cell oxidation.

Sources of vitamin A (carotenoids) include the following:

- Bright orange vegetables like carrots, sweet potatoes, and pumpkin

- Tomatoes and tomato products, red sweet pepper

- Leafy greens such as spinach, collards, turnip greens, kale, beet and mustard greens, green leaf lettuce, and romaine

- Orange fruits like mango, cantaloupe, apricots, and red or pink grapefruit

Sources of vitamin C include these fruits and vegetables:

- Citrus fruits and juices, kiwifruit, strawberries, guava, papaya, and cantaloupe

- Broccoli, peppers, tomatoes, cabbage (especially Chinese cabbage), Brussels sprouts, and potatoes

- Leafy greens such as romaine, turnip greens, and spinach

Sources of vitamin E include these:

- Avocadoes

- Green leafy vegetables

Sources of folate include the following:

- Cooked dry beans and peas

- Oranges and orange juice

- Deep-green leaves like spinach and mustard greens

Sources of potassium include these:

- Baked white or sweet potatoes, cooked greens (such as spinach), winter (orange) squash

- Bananas, plantains, many dried fruits, oranges and orange juice, cantaloupe, and honeydew melons
- Cooked dry beans
- Soybeans (green and mature)
- Tomato products (sauce, paste, purée)
- Beet greens

Tips from 5 to 9 A Day

Here are great tips adapted from the national 5 to 9 A Day campaign on adding fruits and vegetables to your diet.

Fruits

For the best nutritional value:

- Make most of your choices whole or cut-up fruit rather than juice, for the benefits dietary fiber provides.
- Select fruits with more potassium often, such as bananas, prunes and prune juice, dried peaches and apricots, cantaloupe, honeydew melon, and orange juice.
- When choosing canned fruits, select fruit canned in 100 percent fruit juice or water rather than syrup.
- When buying applesauce, select the no-sugar-added variety.
- Vary your fruit choices. Fruits differ in nutrient content.

The following lists some sample options during meals:

- At breakfast, top your cereal with bananas or peaches; add blueberries to pancakes; drink 100 percent orange or grapefruit juice. Or try a fruit mixed with low-fat or fat-free yogurt.
- At lunch, pack a tangerine, banana, or grapes to eat, or choose fruits from a salad bar. Individual containers of fruits such as peaches or applesauce are easy and convenient.

- At dinner, add crushed pineapple to coleslaw, or include mandarin oranges or grapes in a tossed salad.

- Make a Waldorf salad, with apples, celery, walnuts, and low-fat dressing.

- Try meat dishes that incorporate fruit, such as chicken with apricots or mango chutney.

- Add fruit like pineapple or peaches to kabobs as part of a barbecue meal.

- For dessert, have baked apples, pears, or a fruit salad.

Make fruit more appealing:

- Many fruits taste great with a dip or dressing. Try low-fat yogurt as a dip for fruits like strawberries or melons.

- Make a fruit smoothie by blending fat-free or low-fat milk or yogurt with fresh or frozen fruit. Try bananas, peaches, strawberries, or other berries.

- Try applesauce as a fat-free substitute for some of the oil when baking cakes.

- For fresh-fruit salads, mix apples, bananas, or pears with acidic fruits like oranges, pineapple, or lemon juice to keep them from turning brown.

- Choose fruit options such as sliced apples, mixed fruit cup, or 100 percent fruit juice that are available in some fast-food restaurants.

InflamWise _____

Be sure to keep fruits and vegetables away from raw meat, poultry, and seafood while shopping, preparing, or storing. This will keep them from being contaminated with E. coli and other bacteria.

InflamWarnings _____

Beware when buying fruit juices. They are often loaded with added sugar (which is one reason why kids love them). But even without additional sugar, 100 percent fruit juices are still high in fruit sugars and, with the exception of vitamin C, they do not have much nutritional value.

It is better to eat whole fresh fruit than to drink fruit juices, which are high in calories and low in fiber. They are also less filling than natural fruits.

However, if you are going to buy fruit juices, choose those that say "no sugar added."

Vegetables

Here are some tips for purchasing vegetables:

◆ Buy fresh vegetables in season. They cost less and are likely to be at their peak flavor.

◆ Stock up on frozen vegetables for quick and easy cooking in the microwave.

◆ Buy vegetables that are easy to prepare. Pick up prewashed bags of salad greens and add baby carrots or grape tomatoes for a salad in minutes. Buy packages of baby carrots or celery sticks for quick snacks.

◆ Use a microwave to quickly "zap" vegetables. Sweet potatoes can be baked quickly this way.

◆ Vary your veggie choices to keep meals interesting.

◆ Try crunchy vegetables, raw or lightly steamed.

For the best nutritional value, select vegetables with more potassium such as sweet potatoes, white beans, tomato products (paste, sauce, and juice), beet greens, soybeans, lima beans, winter squash, spinach, lentils, kidney beans, and split peas.

Sauces or seasonings can add calories, fat, and sodium to vegetables, so follow these tips:

◆ Prepare more foods from fresh ingredients to lower sodium intake. Most sodium in the food supply comes from packaged or processed foods.

◆ Buy canned vegetables labeled "no salt added." If you want to add a little salt, it will likely be less than the amount in the regular canned product.

When you are planning meals keep in mind the following:

◆ Plan some meals around a vegetable main dish, such as a vegetable stir-fry or soup. Then add other foods to complement it.

◆ Try a main dish salad for lunch. Go light on the salad dressing.

◆ Include a green salad with your dinner every night.

◆ Shred carrots or zucchini into meatloaf, casseroles, quick breads, and muffins.

◆ Include chopped vegetables in pasta sauce or lasagna.

♦ Order a veggie pizza with toppings such as mushrooms, green peppers, and onions, and ask for extra veggies.

♦ Use puréed, cooked vegetables such as potatoes to thicken stews, soups, and gravies. These add flavor, nutrients, and texture.

♦ Grill vegetable kabobs as part of a barbecue meal. Try tomatoes, mushrooms, green peppers, and onions.

Make vegetables more appealing by following these tips:

♦ Many vegetables taste great with a dip or dressing. Try a low-fat salad dressing with raw broccoli, red and green peppers, celery sticks, or cauliflower.

♦ Add color to salads by adding baby carrots, shredded red cabbage, or spinach leaves. Include in-season vegetables for variety through the year.

♦ Include cooked dry beans or peas in flavorful mixed dishes, such as chili or minestrone soup.

♦ Decorate plates or serving dishes with vegetable slices.

♦ Keep a bowl of cut-up vegetables in a see-through container in the refrigerator. Carrot and celery sticks are traditional, but consider broccoli florettes, cucumber slices, or red or green pepper strips.

Grilling Fruits and Vegetables

Grilling fruits and vegetables is a healthful addition to summer barbecues. Grilling summer produce brings out their flavor.

Grill fruits and vegetables as a main dish or a side dish. Grill fruits for an elegant dessert (serve with low-fat frozen yogurt).

Learning to grill produce is easy. If your fruits and vegetables are too small to put on a grill, try using heavy-duty foil or a reusable foil baking pan.

The following are instructions on how to grill fruits and vegetables:

♦ Slice fruit in half and remove pits and cores, if any. Grill with pulp side down to start, then turn over.

♦ Sprinkle a small amount of brown sugar on fruit after grilling if you want a little extra sweetness.

◆ Fruits generally take 3 to 5 minutes to cook. Thinly sliced fruit may take less time. Thicker pieces of fruit, such as halved peaches or pears, may require a little more time. Keep in mind that fruit can burn easily because of its sugar content, so watch it closely.

◆ Cut vegetables into ½-inch slices or large chunks and baste with a light salad dressing, or brush them with canola or olive oil. Grill until tender, turning only once.

◆ Fast-grilling vegetables take about 5 to 7 minutes to cook. These include asparagus, broccoli, baby carrots, eggplant, okra, onion slices, pepper chunks, strips of summer squash, and tomato wedges. Root vegetables, such as beets, winter squash, potatoes and sweet potatoes, take about 20 to 45 minutes to cook, depending on whether they're whole, halved, or cut in slices. Wrap these types of vegetables in foil with a drizzle of oil and a sprinkling of spices and herbs.

Here are some ideas for grilling fruits:

◆ Cut fruit, such as apples, pears, and peaches, into chunks, brush lightly with canola oil, and place on skewers or wrap in foil before grilling. A sprinkle of cinnamon before grilling adds a flavorful touch.

◆ Slice bananas with their peels lengthwise and brush the cut side with canola oil. Place cut side down on the grill and cook until lightly browned, about 2 minutes. Turn and grill until the bananas begin to pull away from the peel, about 2 to 4 minutes more.

◆ Sprinkle brown sugar onto ½-inch-thick pineapple slices. Grill the slices, turning a few times, until browned, about 5 minutes.

◆ Brush pear wedges with lemon juice and grill, turning a few times, until they begin to brown, about 2 to 4 minutes. Add to a mixed green salad.

Try these ideas for cooking vegetables on the grill:

◆ Marinate a large portobello mushroom in French or Italian dressing—or make your own dressing with 1½ tablespoons balsamic vinegar, 1½ tablespoons olive oil, a clove of minced garlic, salt, and pepper—and grill it like a burger. Serve on a bun or alone.

◆ Soak ears of corn in water for 30 minutes, then grill in the husk for 15 to 20 minutes. Remove the silk before grilling.

◆ Cut vegetables such as squash, peppers, onions, and mushrooms into equal-sized pieces. Place on a skewer with shrimp or chunks of turkey breast. Brush with fresh fruit juice or broth and grill. These can also be wrapped in aluminum foil before grilling.

◆ Cut tomatoes in half crosswise, brush with canola or olive oil, and add salt, pepper, and your favorite spices. Wrap in foil and grill sliced side up for 6 to 8 minutes.

◆ Cut a head of radicchio into quarters and brush with a mixture of orange juice, olive oil, and orange zest. Grill until tender, about 8 to 10 minutes.

Here are some ideas for grilled desserts:

◆ Try grilled fruit instead of fat-laden ice cream or cake. The dry heat of grilling intensifies and caramelizes the natural sugars in fruit. Favorite desserts include halves or slices of apricots, peaches, plums, and nectarines. For something different, try sliced apples, figs, and pears. A banana cooked slowly in its peel results in a custardlike delicacy—perfect for the end of a meal.

◆ Grill slices of low-fat angel food cake for 1 to 3 minutes or until golden brown on both sides. Top with chilled strawberries, blueberries, or raspberries.

◆ Make cantaloupe kabobs. Brush with a mixture of honey, butter, and chopped mint. Cook 3 to 4 minutes, turning the fruit to grill each side.

◆ Fill peach halves with blueberries and sprinkle with brown sugar and lemon juice. Wrap in aluminum foil and grill for 15 to 20 minutes, turning once.

The Least You Need to Know

◆ Eating fruits and vegetables can lower your CRP levels.

◆ Eating produce fights many diseases, including macular degeneration.

◆ Produce is a great source of fiber.

◆ You can prepare fruits and vegetables in a way that appeals to everyone in your family.

Chapter 11

Putting It into Action: Eliminate Processed and Refined Foods

In This Chapter

◆ Because the perils of processed and refined foods

◆ Understand the connection between processed and refined foods and insulin resistance

◆ Learn how to replace some foods with organic foods

◆ Discover the miracle of water

The final principle of the anti-inflammation diet is to eliminate processed and refined foods from your diet. After the subtraction of these additives, chemicals, and empty calories, you will enjoy eating primarily the health-promoting fats, lean proteins, grains, fruits, and vegetables that are the framework of the diet.

In this chapter, we cover the numerous substances that are at the center of the trouble in processed and refined foods. They include refined sugar, refined flour, salt, additives, and preservatives. We also cover the dangers of glucose intolerance—a typical problem resulting from eating too many processed and refined foods.

The Perils of Processed and Refined Foods

The final principle of the anti-inflammation diet is based, in part, on research conducted by the World Health Organization (WHO). In 2003 WHO published a report by an international team of top scientists urging people to cut their intake of processed foods, which are often high in saturated fats, sugar, and salt. The researchers said eating more fruits and vegetables (Principle #6 of the anti-inflammation diet) and exercising more were the best ways to protect against chronic health problems.

Did You Know?

About 90 percent of the money Americans spend on food is used to buy processed food.

The statement was an incredible event: the highly respected WHO setting an official policy telling the world to stay away from processed foods.

Eating processed and refined foods means eating empty calories—and it usually means eating lots of trans fats, salt, sugar, and toxins, as well. What you don't get is much nutrition.

Processed and refined foods are everywhere. They include the bacon you eat for breakfast, the festive birthday cake you pick up at the grocery store for your 2-year-old, and the soda you drink every day at 4:00 to "get through" to dinner. Examples of processed or refined foods are frozen meals, canned goods, prepackaged meals, fried foods, cakes, cookies, canned biscuits, chips, breakfast bars, toaster treats, white flour, white bread, white rice, white pasta, sodas, juice with sugar, margarine, mayonnaise, and any foods containing hydrogenated oils.

Processed and refined foods have much longer "shelf lives" than whole foods, which makes them appealing to grocery stores and consumers because they can stay on their shelves for months and even years and not spoil. In fact, almost anything that could spoil has been refined right out of these foods.

Processed Foods and Insulin Resistance

The refined grains and sugars in processed foods create problems with glucose tolerance. In whole foods, starches are complex and your body has to break them down to turn them into the glucose your body needs. The process takes a while, which is the way your body was made to work.

In contrast, refined grains and sugars are already broken down. Zap, and your body has absorbed them with lightning speed. (This is where the phrase "sugar rush" comes from.)

When refined grains and sugars enter your system, your blood and cells are almost instantly swamped with glucose. Your body thinks "Emergency!" and insulin sweeps in to mop up the glucose, which it gets rid of by turning it into fat.

The process is particularly bad for us if we do it over and over again by eating highly processed and refined breakfasts, lunches, dinners, snacks, and drinks. Over time, our bodies stop responding to insulin, leading to a condition called *insulin resistance*. Insulin resistance, in turn, leads to metabolic syndrome—and unchecked and silent inflammation.

 InflamWise

The phrase "refined foods" has an interesting origin. It originates with the refined people (that is, the wealthy ones) whose staff hand-sifted whole wheat to create pure white flour. Only very wealthy, refined people could afford this process. The peasants, who were unrefined, ate whole grains.

def•i•ni•tion

Insulin resistance is a silent condition that increases the chances of developing diabetes and heart disease. If you have insulin resistance, your muscle, fat, and liver cells do not use insulin efficiently. Your body tries to keep up with the demand for it by producing more. This is the responsibility of your pancreas. But it isn't up to the task, and excess sugar builds up in your bloodstream.

Many people with insulin resistance have high levels of blood sugar and insulin in their blood at the same time.

The Glycemic Index

The glycemic index (GI) is a ranking of carbohydrates on a scale from 0 to 100. Foods with a high GI are rapidly digested and absorbed, resulting in high blood sugar. Low-GI foods are slowly digested and absorbed, causing gradual rises in blood sugar and insulin levels. They are good for health.

Low GI diets:

◆ Improve glucose levels.

◆ Help control appetite and delay hunger.

◆ Reduce insulin levels and insulin resistance.

Studies at the Harvard School of Public Health show that the risks of diabetes and coronary heart disease are connected to GI levels. In other words, the more foods you eat with high GI levels, the higher your risk of these diseases. In 1999, WHO recommended that people in industrialized countries base their diets on low GI foods. That pretty much means eliminating a lot of refined and processed foods. In fact, the biggest GI offenders include white bread, bagels, crackers, cornflakes, and instant potatoes. Even rice cakes have high GI levels.

How to Stay Away from High GI Foods

There are a number of resources for tracking the GI levels of foods, including the Internet. But in truth, figuring out which foods are "high GI" and "low GI" is complicated, and may not be that beneficial. Strangely enough, some processed foods, such as candy bars and pizza, have low GIs because the fat in them keeps them from being digested and absorbed quickly.

InflamWise

There are two bases used for determining GI levels—white bread or glucose—so if you decide to use a glycemic index, make sure that you know which database you are using.

We suggest the following: when it comes to your diet, keep refined sugars and grains to a minimum and you will most likely keep your GI in a normal range.

Highly Processed and Refined Foods

The ingredient list for refined and processed foods goes something like this:

◆ Lots of salt

◆ Lots of refined sugar

◆ Artificial flavors to taste

◆ Artificial colors also to taste (this one visual)

◆ Some other additives

◆ Some preservatives

◆ Maybe some refined flour

This list used to include bad-for-you fats, but their use in processed foods has lessened because they now have to be listed on product labels.

There are a number of processed and refined offenders. Here are just a few examples:

◆ Donuts have no virtues beyond their taste. They are made from processed white flour, fried in bad fats, and covered with sugar. They even have a fair amount of sodium.

◆ Refined grain products such as white bread, crackers, pasta, cookies, and cakes have limited nutritional value and no fiber, and virtually all vitamins and minerals are destroyed in the refining process. (Use whole-grain versions of these products instead.)

◆ Bacon, sausage, ham, and lunch meats that contain nitrates and nitrites, which are toxic chemicals that can develop into cancer-causing nitrosamines. And do we even need to mention that they are often vessels of saturated fat and sodium?

◆ Microwave popcorn has replaced stove-top popping in vegetable oil. It is usually loaded with trans fats, unless the package says "trans-fat-free" on it.

◆ Canned foods have generally had all the good processed right out of them and then they have been bombarded by additives. They are also usually high in sodium.

Here is a list of some of the chemicals in two popular types of soup, chicken bouillon granules and vegetable beef: sodium phosphate, monosodium glutamate, caramel color, potassium chloride, lactic acid, disodium inosinate and disodium guanylate, tricalcium phosphate, alpha tocopherol, BHA preservative, propyl gallate, citric acid, and BHT preservative. Sounds a lot like a recipe for bug killer, doesn't it?

Salt

Food processors use *salt* (*sodium* chloride) because it helps prevent spoiling and extends shelf life. It draws water out of the food and helps prevent bacteria from growing. It also kills some bacteria; adds flavor to food; makes food seem thicker; increases sweetness in soft drinks, cookies, cakes, and other products; covers up the taste of chemicals; and can keep foods dry. High salt intake has been scientifically linked to high blood pressure, but there are presently no recommendations on how much salt a day is the best for health.

The DASH eating plan, which is clinically proven to significantly reduce blood pressure, recommends lowering your intake of salt. (DASH stands for Dietary Approaches to Stop Hypertension. The plan, developed by the National Institutes of Health, is

def•i•ni•tion

The terms **salt** and **sodium**, often used interchangeably, are not the same. Sodium is an element that joins with chlorine to form sodium chloride, which we know as table salt. Sodium occurs naturally in most foods, but salt is the most common source of sodium in our foods.

discussed extensively in Chapter 18.) It bases its diet on 2,400 milligrams of sodium per day and suggests further lowering salt intake to 1,500 milligrams per day. Twenty-four hundred milligrams of sodium equals about 6 grams, or 1 teaspoon, of table salt; 1,500 milligrams of sodium equals about 4 grams, or ⅔ teaspoon, of table salt. To give a little perspective on these amounts: 1½ ounces of processed cheese has 600 milligrams of salt, and the crackers that go with it have another 1,100 milligrams of salt (based on 3.5 ounces of saltines).

Here are some other examples of salt in processed foods per 3.5-ounce serving:

Bacon, cooked: 1,021

Bacon, Canadian: 2,500

Beans, lima (regular canned): 236

Beans, canned with pork and tomato sauce: 463

Beef hash, canned: 540

Beef, dried: 4,300

Bouillon cubes: 24,000

Canned soups: 350 to 450

Cereal, rice flakes: 987

Cereal, wheat flakes: 1,000

Cheese, cottage: 406

Cheese, cream: 296

Cheese, mozzarella: 373

Cheese, Parmesan: 1,862

Cocoa, processed: 717

Cookies, fig bars: 252

Cookies, oatmeal: 170

Cookies, plain: 365

Crabmeat, canned: 1,000

Crackers, graham: 670

Doughnuts: 500

Margarine: 987

Olives, green: 2,400

Peanut butter: 607

Pickles, dill: 1,428

Pickles, relish, sweet: 712

Popcorn, salted with oil: 1,940

Pork, cured ham: 930

Pork, canned ham: 1,100

Pretzels: 1,680

Sausage, pork: 958

Sausage, frankfurter: 1,100

Sausage, bologna: 1,300

Tomato ketchup: 1,042

Source: Washington University School of Medicine.

Sugar

What can we say about sugar? It tastes heavenly. It kills. Detecting how much sugar is in a product takes some serious detective work.

Added sugars are sugars and syrups that are added to foods or beverages during processing or preparation. This does not include naturally occurring sugars, such as those that occur in milk and fruits.

Foods that contain most of the added sugars in American diets are:

- Regular soft drinks
- Candy
- Cakes
- Cookies
- Pies
- Fruit drinks, such as fruitades and fruit punch
- Milk-based desserts and products, such as ice cream, sweetened yogurt, and sweetened milk
- Flour-based products, such as sweet rolls and cinnamon toast

> **Did You Know?**
>
> According to the National Institutes of Health, the average American eats about 147 pounds of sugar a year.

Typically, when ingredients are listed on a product, they must be listed from the largest amount down to the smallest amount found in that product. Do not be fooled into thinking there is only a little sugar in an item if it is not listed near the beginning. Often you will find three or four of the following aliases in the ingredient listing:

- Brown sugar
- Corn syrup
- Corn sweetener
- Dextrose
- Fructose
- Fruit juice concentrates
- High-fructose corn syrup
- Honey
- Invert sugar
- Lactose
- Maltose
- Maltodextrin
- Malt syrup
- Molasses
- Raw sugar
- Sucrose

- Sugar

- Syrup

- White grape juice

If three or four of these are on an ingredient list for a product, the item is probably mostly sugar.

Toxin Watch List

The Center for Science in the Public Interest (CSPI) is an advocacy organization for nutrition and health, food safety, alcohol policy, and sound science. Some of the additives that they recommend avoiding are sodium nitrite, saccharin, olestra, and artificial coloring. CSPI points out that these ingredients should be avoided anyway because they are used primarily in foods of little nutritional value. Here are some details:

- Sodium nitrite and sodium nitrate. Used in bacon, ham, frankfurters, luncheon meats, smoked fish, and corned beef, these preservatives are used to prevent the growth of bacteria that cause botulism poisoning. In addition, sodium nitrite keeps meats looking red and "healthy."

  Their danger? They can form cancer-causing substances in the stomach called nitrosamines. Happily, the use of nitrite and nitrate has decreased greatly over the last decade.

- Saccharin. This sweetener is in diet products such as soft drinks, or it can be found in packets next to sugar. A popular brand is Sweet 'N Low. It is 350 times sweeter than sugar and is used in dietetic foods or as a tabletop sugar substitute. Many studies have been done on saccharin, with some showing a correlation with cancer (especially bladder cancer) and others showing no such correlation. However, for now it is probably wise to avoid saccharin and other artificial sweeteners until more testing has been done.

- Artificial colorings. Most artificial colorings are synthetic chemicals. Because colorings are used mostly in junk foods loaded with empty calories, they should be avoided. Some colorings can cause hyperactivity in children.

- Olestra is a fake fat that seems like a dieter's dream. It is sometimes used in potato chips and other snack foods. Although it tastes like fat, its molecules are too big for the body to digest, and it does not turn to fat but goes right through your digestive system. However, in addition to frequently causing diarrhea, when it leaves your body, olestra takes with it many health-promoting substances, such as the antioxidant carotenoids.

CSPI also warns that the following additives in foods may cause allergic reactions or other problems for some people. For example, sulfite and sulfur dioxide can be a serious problem for people with asthma. Be wary of the following ingredients:

- Artificial colorings
- Yellow 5
- Artificial and natural flavoring
- Aspartame (Nutrasweet)
- Beta-carotene
- Caffeine
- Carmine; cochineal
- Casein
- Gum tragacanth
- HVP (hydrolyzed vegetable protein)
- Lactose
- MSG (monosodium glutamate)
- Mycoprotein
- Quinine
- Sodium bisulfite
- Sulfites
- Sulfur dioxide

The Virtues of Organic Foods

One of the options for avoiding processed foods is to purchase organic foods if they fit into your budget. Even mainstream groceries have organic sections in their supermarkets these days.

What does it mean when a food is advertised as organic? The U.S. Department of Agriculture issues a national seal certifying that the food meets certain guidelines. Only foods certified as at least 95 percent organic are allowed to carry the official "USDA organic" seal.

Organic food is produced without using most conventional pesticides, fertilizers made with synthetic ingredients or sewage sludge, bioengineering, or ionizing radiation.

Organic farms need to prove that these materials have not been used for at least three years. Before a product can be labeled organic, a government official inspects the farm where the food is grown to make sure the farmer is following all the rules necessary to meet USDA organic standards.

Companies that handle or process organic food before it gets to your local supermarket or restaurant must be certified, too.

Under these rules, organic foods belong to one of four categories:

1. Food that is 100 percent organic may carry the "USDA organic" label and say "100 percent organic."

2. Food that is at least 95 percent organic may carry the seal.

3. Food that is at least 70 percent organic may list the organic ingredients on the front of the package.

4. If a product is less than 70 percent organic, the organic ingredients may be listed on the side of the package but the product cannot say "organic" on the front.

InflamWise

You may see labels such as "natural," "free-range," and "hormone-free" on food labels. However, don't confuse these terms with "organic." Only food labeled "organic" has been certified as meeting USDA organic standards.

Look for the word "organic" and a small sticker version of the USDA organic seal on vegetables or pieces of fruit, or on the sign above the organic produce display. The word "organic" and the seal may also appear on packages of meat, cartons of milk or eggs, cheese, and other single-ingredient foods. Use of the seal is voluntary.

Organic food is now big business. Organic food sales in the United States are increasing by about 20 percent a year and were over $20 billion in 2005.

Avoiding Pesticides

One approach is to reserve your organic shopping dollars for those types of foods that are apt to be most contaminated with toxins. Nonorganically grown spinach, for example, contains more pesticide residue than almost any other fruit or vegetable.

The nonprofit research organization Environmental Working Group (EWG) found that more than half of the total dietary risk from pesticides is concentrated in just 12 crops. The pesticides that were found in these foods are classified by the Environmental Protection Agency (EPA) as "probable human carcinogens, nervous system poisons, and endocrine system disrupters."

According to EWG, here are the 12 most contaminated foods:

- Strawberries
- Green and red bell peppers
- Spinach
- Cherries (U.S.)

- ◆ Peaches
- ◆ Cantaloupe (Mexican)
- ◆ Celery
- ◆ Apples

- ◆ Apricots
- ◆ Green beans
- ◆ Grapes (Chilean)
- ◆ Cucumbers

You may want to reserve your organic shopping dollars for these foods or, if you do not have access to an organic market, avoid eating them.

Tips for Finding and Buying Organic Foods

The following are tips on how to buy organic foods:

- ◆ To find organic food in your community, look for organic associations in your state. On the Internet type the name of your state and the word "organic" into a search engine and see what pops up.

- ◆ Check out your local farmers' market. Farmers' markets are great sources of affordable, local organic produce.

- ◆ Buy a share in a community-supported agriculture program. When you buy a share in a community-supported agriculture (CSA) program, you pay a portion of a local farm's operating expenses. In return, you receive weekly boxes of fresh fruits and vegetables in the upcoming harvest.

- ◆ Join an organic co-op. An organic food cooperative is a member-owned business that provides groceries and other products to its members at a discount.

- ◆ Buy organic produce at the peak buying season and freeze them. Be sure to eat them within 6 months.

Cut Back on All Soft Drinks

Today the average American consumes over 240 pints of soft drinks a year—over 30 gallons. Jokingly referred to by nutritionists as "liquid candy," we all know the sugary form of soda pop is bad for us. But so is diet soda. The chemicals in both types of soft drinks include artificial flavorings, artificial color additives and dyes, acidifying agents, buffering agents, viscosity-producing agents, foaming agents, and preservatives. One of these additives is phosphoric acid. Through a chain of events, phosphoric acid is responsible for calcium being leached from our bones.

Did You Know?

Phosphoric acid is used to acidify foods and beverages such as colas. It provides a tangy taste, and is available cheaply and in large quantities. It mimics more expensive natural seasonings such as ginger, lemons, and limes. It also helps keep the carbonated bubbles from going flat.

Phosphoric acid can also neutralize the hydrochloric acid in our stomachs, which we need to help us digest our food and use its nutrients.

The Miracle of Water

This is as good a time as any to laud the benefits of water and its role in a health-promoting diet. Replace all those high-sugar and high-chemical drinks with water.

Water makes up more than two thirds of the weight of the human body. In fact, the human brain is made up of 95 percent water. Water is key to keep your body running smoothly. And tap water is virtually free. Make a conscious effort to keep yourself hydrated and make water your beverage of choice.

How much water should we drink? The truth is that no one knows for sure. There is general agreement among experts that the old rule that we should drink eight 8-ounce glasses per day is not based on science. We do know that adults lose between 2 to 3 quarts of water per day by way of normal body functions. But if you are active and/or live in a warm climate, you will lose more. If you are one of these people, you need to drink more water. Some fruit juices and green tea can count as fluid intake, but you cannot count coffee or alcohol. They have mild diuretic effects.

One rule of thumb is to drink one cup of water for every 20 pounds of body weight if you are sedentary. Increase this amount if you are more active. However, the best indicator that you are drinking enough water is when your urine comes out pale yellow to clear. A dark yellow color is a sign that your body is dehydrated.

InflamWise

If you drink water from a bottle, thoroughly clean or replace the bottle often. Every time you drink, bacteria from your mouth contaminates water in the bottle. If you use a bottle repeatedly, make sure that the bottle is designed for reuse. To keep it clean, all you have to do is wash your container in hot, soapy water or run it through a dishwasher before refilling it.

Organic Treats for Kids

Here are some tips on choosing nutritious snacks for kids.

- ◆ Select baked potato chips instead of fried potato chips.

- ◆ Many microwave popcorns are also high in harmful fats. Look for the products that say "trans-fat-free."

- ◆ Yes, nuts are high in fat, but the fat is actually a good one. Nuts are also high in protein and essential vitamins and minerals.

- ◆ Put together a snack mix of peanuts and raisins. You also might want to add in some 70 percent cocoa chocolate chips. (The package should say that the chips contain 70 percent cocoa.) Skip the high-fat items such as granola and breakfast bars.

- ◆ Sunflower seeds are high in energy, fiber, and protein. Again, they're high in fat, but most of it is the good kind.

- ◆ Kids love frozen fruit bars. Make sure that they have no added sugars. The best have chunks of real fruit such as orange, pineapple, peach, and banana, to name a few.

- ◆ Try keeping a bowl of grapes in the freezer for an unusual treat. Kids of all ages love to pop them in their mouths.

Fun Recipes for Kids (and Adults, Too!)

Ants on a Log

2 celery sticks

6 tsp. natural peanut butter

2 tsp. raisins

Wash the celery and cut it into pieces (each piece should be about 5 inches long). Spread peanut butter in U-shaped part of celery, from one end to the other. Press raisins gently into peanut butter.

Banana Push-Ups

1¼ large bananas, cut up

⅓ cup nonfat dry milk

⅔ cup plain yogurt

¼ lb. frozen pineapple or orange juice concentrate

⅔ cup water

8 small paper cups

Combine bananas, dry milk, yogurt, juice concentrate, and water in a blender and blend until foamy. Pour into paper cups and freeze. Push up from bottom of the cup to eat.

Frozen Banana Pops

½ cup 70 percent cocoa chocolate chips

2 TB. honey

¼ cup natural peanut butter

2 TB. nonfat milk

4 medium firm bananas, cut in half

⅓ cup finely chopped nuts

8 wooden popsicle sticks

In a small heavy saucepan, over low heat, melt chocolate chips and honey, stirring constantly. Add peanut butter, stirring until smooth. Remove from heat and stir in milk.

Peel bananas and insert wooden sticks into thickest end.

Spoon chocolate mixture over bananas to coat or dip bananas into mixture if possible. Roll coated banana in chopped nuts and place on a wax paper–lined cookie sheet.

Chocolate-Dipped Strawberries

2 large 70 percent cocoa dark chocolate bars

12 large fresh organic strawberries with stems

Wash and dry the strawberries, leaving stems on. Break chocolate into small pieces and place in microwave-safe bowl. Heat in microwave oven on high for 30 seconds. (Some microwaves may take a little longer.) Holding by stems, dip each strawberry. Place on wax paper to cool.

Yogurt Pops

1 (8 oz.) container of your favorite flavor of yogurt

Small paper cups

Wooden popsicle sticks

Plastic wrap

Pour yogurt into paper cups. Fill them almost to the top. Stretch a small piece of plastic wrap across the top of each cup. Using the popsicle stick, poke a hole in the plastic wrap. Stand the stick straight up in the center of the cup. Put the cups in the freezer until the yogurt is frozen solid. Remove the plastic wrap, peel away the paper cup.

Peanut Butter Play Dough

2 cups natural peanut butter

2 cups powdered milk

3 TB. honey

Mix together peanut butter, powdered milk, and honey. Add more powdered milk, one tablespoon at a time, if it is too sticky.

The Least You Need to Know

- Avoid processed and refined foods to prevent insulin resistance.

- Read labels carefully to find out how much sugar is really in a product.

- To cut back on salt and to stay away from toxins, avoid processed and refined foods.

- Buy organic foods in place of high-pesticide foods.

- Replace sodas with water.

Chapter 12

Through the Life Cycle

In This Chapter

- ◆ How many calories you need during your life cycle
- ◆ Understand the concerns about the childhood obesity epidemic
- ◆ Learn about the Tufts pyramid
- ◆ See the nutritional guidelines for seniors

Our nutritional needs change throughout our lives. For example, we would not expect a 20-year-old woman to eat the same things that she did at age 2. And we should not expect her to eat the same things at age 70 that she does now.

Regardless of your age, it is important to stay within a healthy calorie range for your age group. This chapter covers the changing nutritional needs of individuals as they grow older and age, with particular focus on the senior years.

Different Ages and Different Nutritional Needs

Our nutritional needs change as we grow up, reach adulthood, and grow older. For example, in a family with a grandparent, mother and father, and two children ages 5 and 15, the daily calorie levels might be something like this:

◆ Granddad, age 72, used to be able to eat anything he wanted and he stayed slim. But he had to give up sweets because these days they seem to go right to his stomach. He eats about 1,700 calories a day.

◆ Mom, age 35, who is very active and walks at least 3 miles a day, should get about 2,200 calories a day, down from the 2,400 she could eat 5 years ago when she was 30. If she eats more she could gain weight. If she eats less she might not have enough energy and nutrients to sustain her active life.

◆ Dad, who is a couch potato, gets to eat more calories: 2,400 to 2,600. (This seems a bit unfair.) But he should step up his activity level to maintain his health.

◆ Brittany, age 15, who is very active, has the same calorie requirement as her mother: 2,400. However, she is aware that if she stops being so active and keeps eating that many calories, she will gain weight.

◆ Tommy, age 5, who can't sit still, should get from 1,600 to 2,000 calories a day. Tommy and his parents have a problem. A lot of his calories come from junk food and not the nutritional sources he needs.

This family represents some of the nutritional needs that change over time. Here is a table of estimates from the prestigious Institute of Medicine (IOM), of the National Academy of Sciences, for how many calories you need depending on your age, gender, and how active you are. In this table:

◆ Sedentary means a lifestyle that includes only the light physical activity associated with typical day-to-day life.

◆ Moderately active means a lifestyle that includes physical activity equivalent to walking about 1.5 to 3 miles per day at 3 to 4 miles per hour, in addition to the light physical activity associated with typical day-to-day life.

◆ Active means a lifestyle that includes physical activity equivalent to walking more than 3 miles per day at 3 to 4 miles per hour, in addition to the light physical activity associated with typical day-to-day life.

As the following table shows, the need for calories varies greatly with age. Trouble occurs when we eat too little or too many calories for our needs. And for Americans, the most frequently occurring problem is eating too many empty calories.

Calories Needed Throughout the Life Cycle

		Activity Level		
Gender	*Age (yrs)*	*Sedentary*	*Moderately Active*	*Active*
Child	2–3	1,000	1,000–1,400	1,000–1,400
Female	4–8	1,200	1,400–1,600	1,400–1,800
	9–13	1,600	1,600–2,000	1,800–2,200
	14–18	1,800	2,000	2,400
	19–30	2,000	2,000–2,200	2,400
	31–50	1,800	2,000	2,200
	51+	1,600	1,800	2,000–2,200
Male	4–8	1,400	1,400–1,600	1,600–2,000
	9–13	1,800	1,800–2,200	2,000–2,600
	14–18	2,200	2,400–2,800	2,800–3,200
	19–30	2,400	2,600–2,800	3,000
	31–50	2,200	2,400–2,600	2,800–3,000
	51+	2,000	2,200–2,400	2,400–2,800

Source: Institute of Medicine Dietary Reference Intakes Macronutrients Report, 2002.

Obesity in Children and Teens

Obesity in kids has reached epidemic levels. Estimates are that 15 percent of kids are overweight and another 15 percent are high risk of becoming overweight. And two thirds of these overweight kids will become overweight adults.

Over the past 3 decades, the childhood obesity rate has more than doubled for preschool children aged 2 to 5 years and adolescents aged 12 to 19 years, and it has more than tripled for children aged 6 to 11 years.

A number of factors may contribute to the rise in childhood obesity:

◆ Kids are walking less and not engaging in as many physical activities as they used to.

◆ There is frequent consumption of convenience foods that are high in calories and fat.

◆ It is costly to purchase wholesome foods such as fruits, vegetables, and other nutritious foods.

◆ There are few opportunities for physical activity at school.

◆ Kids now spend more time watching television or playing computer and video games rather than enjoying physical activity.

The Risk of Disease

Many people believe that bad nutrition only takes its toll on adults. Not true. A number of studies have shown that diabetes is on the rise in children, and a population-based study found that approximately 60 percent of obese children aged 5 to 10 years had at least one cardiovascular disease risk factor—such as elevated total cholesterol, triglycerides, insulin, or blood pressure—and 25 percent had two or more CVD risk factors.

A major reason why obesity in children is increasing is easily stated in two words: junk food. For example, the authors of the IOM's report on childhood obesity point out that by the time children are 14 years old, 52 percent of boys and 32 percent of girls are drinking three or more 8-ounce servings of soda a day.

The Power of Advertising

Part of the reason for children's love of junk food comes from the fact that they are bombarded with advertising promoting empty calories. The IOM found the following:

> The food and beverage industries spend $10 billion to $12 billion annually marketing directly to children and youth. The average child views more than 40,000 TV commercials each year and more than half of TV ads directed at kids promote high-calorie foods and beverages such as candy, snack foods, fast foods, soft drinks, and sweetened breakfast cereals. In addition, the entertainment industry promotes many products that encourage sedentary behaviors.

Without question, children and teens can benefit from the anti-inflammation diet and lifestyle. Cutting out junk food (a.k.a. processed and refined foods), eating health-promoting foods, and getting adequate exercise can help nip obesity and its inflammation-related problems before they get out of control. (And, of course, not smoking is critical.)

Nutrition and Aging

Former Prime Minister of Israel Golda Meir and noted anthropologist Margaret Mead are both credited with the remark: "Old age is like flying through a storm. Once you're aboard, there's nothing you can do." Whoever said it was wrong. There are many things you can do during later life to ease the aging process and prevent inflammation. Along with exercise and weight control, diet is at the top of the list.

One of the least understood concepts about aging is that as we grow older, our energy requirements decrease. At the same time, when we are older we need high-quality protein to maintain our muscles. This is particularly important if illness strikes or we are inactive.

Aging affects the absorption, utilization, and excretion of nutrients. And it is not always easy to eat well. With age people lose some of their ability to taste, smell, and see. Additional problems can occur:

- Difficulty preparing food due to illness, arthritis, immobility, loss of sight, or other problems

- A similar difficulty with shopping and carrying groceries

- Loss of teeth, making it difficult to chew

- Not enough money to buy the food you need

- A loss of interest in food due to illness, medications, grief, or related problems

Nutrient Needs

Although there is a lot we don't know about aging and nutrition, there are some things that are important to understand so that you can make adjustments in your daily habits.

First, your body may not be able to use food as well as it did when you were younger. Therefore, there is a need for more nutrients. At the same time, as you age, you need to cut down on calories or you will gain weight. So nutrient-dense foods, which give more bang for your calories, are very important.

Nutrient-dense foods are chock-full of vitamins and minerals, but low in calories. They include fruits, vegetables, whole grains, low-fat dairy products, and lean protein. (In other words, the foods found in the seven principles of the anti-inflammation diet.)

Second, calcium may be a concern for you for several reasons. Your stomach may secrete less hydrochloric acid, which may reduce the amount of calcium you can absorb. Hormonal changes can alter your body's ability to absorb calcium and you may lose calcium through your kidneys. In addition, lactose intolerance may cause you to lose the ability to digest lactose, the sugar in milk.

If you are lactose intolerant, you may want to experiment with different approaches to eating and drinking dairy products, because it is important to get enough calcium. Some tips are:

♦ Drink small amounts of milk at one time.

♦ Drink milk with foods.

♦ Try milks processed especially for people with lactose problems.

♦ You may be able to tolerate some milk products better than others, such as buttermilk, yogurt, and acidophilus milk.

♦ You might want to try the enzyme lactase, which changes the lactose in regular milk to a type of sugar that might be friendlier to your digestion.

♦ Other sources of calcium include collard, mustard and turnip greens, broccoli, pinto beans, and canned salmon and sardines (with bones).

InflamWarnings

Don't take iron supplements unless your doctor specifically recommends it. Too much iron can damage your organs.

Third, iron is very important during older age, particularly for people who have been told that they are anemic or have "low blood." But it is also difficult to get enough in the food you eat. Not many foods have significant levels of iron. The best sources are meat, whole grain breads and cereals, dry beans, and some fruits and vegetables. And remember that old iron stew pot? You may want to get it out of storage. Cooking with iron utensils helps to get iron into your system.

Fourth, with age many people lose their sense of thirst, but they actually need to drink more water, not less. Older people dehydrate faster than when they were younger. Try to drink six to eight glasses of water a day, even if you don't feel thirsty. And don't drink less water to decrease the number of trips you take to the bathroom. Water is very important for good health.

Here are some other important tips and guidelines for older people:

◆ During older age, you need higher levels of calcium and vitamin D than when you were younger to reduce the risk of osteoporosis, fractures, and disability. The American Medical Women's Association (AMWA) recommends 700 to 800 International Units of vitamin D for women and men over age 50 to reduce the risk of bone fracture by 25 percent.

   However, nutritionists from Tufts recommend taking a little less calcium and vitamin D (see further on in this chapter). You may want to discuss these recommendations with a nutritionist, doctor, or other health-care provider. Whichever recommendation you choose to use, the point is to make sure that you get plenty of vitamin D to protect your bones. Nonfat milk provides an excellent source of calcium and vitamin D. Nonfat dairy products offer the best source of calcium. The best dietary food source of vitamin D is oily fish.

◆ Many of us get our vitamin D from the sun. However, the skin of older adults does not synthesize vitamin D as well as that of younger people. In addition, if you are housebound or live in an institution, you may not receive sufficient amounts of vitamin D.

◆ A new study suggests that a diet rich in foods containing vitamin E may help protect some people against Alzheimer's disease (AD). The study was also noteworthy for its finding that vitamin E in the form of supplements was not associated with a reduction in the risk of AD.

◆ A diet with a high intake of beta-carotene, vitamins C and E, and zinc is associated with a substantially reduced risk of age-related macular degeneration in elderly persons (see Chapter 2).

◆ As mentioned in Chapter 3, studies at Tufts University suggest that a diet rich in whole grains can help prevent metabolic syndrome in older people. Results showed that as whole-grain intake increased, blood sugar levels lowered.

◆ Eating more fiber might help you avoid intestinal problems such as constipation, diverticulosis, and diverticulitis. It might also lower cholesterol and blood sugar and help you have regular bowel movements. If you are not used to eating a lot of fiber, add more fiber to your diet *slowly* to avoid stomach problems. The best source of this fiber is food, rather than dietary supplements.

◆ Most people eat a lot more sodium than they need. If you are over age 50, aim for 1,500 milligrams of sodium—about ⅔ of a teaspoon of table salt. That includes all the sodium you get in your food and drink, not just what you add when cooking or eating. If your doctor tells you to use less salt, cut back on salty snacks and processed foods.

Try adding spices, herbs, and lemon juice to replace sodium and add flavor to your food. Also make sure your diet is rich in foods containing potassium. That will help counter the effects of salt on your blood pressure. Some foods that have a lot of potassium are leafy green vegetables, fruit from vines such as tomatoes, bananas, and root vegetables.

At the same time, do not go overboard with foods that contain potassium. While it is an important nutrient, in large doses, particularly in combination with some medications, it can be dangerous and even lethal.

◆ Because your sense of taste and smell may not work as well as you get older, you may not always be able to tell if foods have gone bad. You might want to date foods in your refrigerator to keep yourself from eating foods that are no longer fresh. If in doubt, throw it out.

Older people should be very careful with certain kinds of foods that need to be well cooked to prevent disease. For example, be sure to fully cook eggs, pork, fish, shellfish, poultry, and hot dogs. You might want to talk to your doctor or a registered dietitian, a specialist trained in nutrition, about foods you should avoid. These might include raw sprouts, some deli meats, and foods that are not pasteurized (heated enough to destroy disease-causing organisms), including some milk products.

At the same time, a number of problems can create hurdles that must be surmounted to get a healthful diet after age 70:

◆ Activity level: If you are a senior you may find that you are cutting back on activities for physical and medical reasons, which can lead to weight gain, which, in turn, can cause a rise in CRP levels.

◆ Metabolism: Every year over the age of 40, metabolism slows down. A decrease in lean body tissue (muscle) and more sedentary lifestyles contribute to the slowing. If you continue to eat the same amount and types of food that you did when you were younger, you're likely to gain weight because you're burning fewer calories. If you are also exercising less, this can cause double trouble.

◆ Taste and appetite: Your senses of taste and smell lessen with age, sometimes making food less interesting. In addition, some medicines can change your sense of taste or make you feel less hungry. Or you need less calories because you aren't as active as you used to be. Sometimes chewing is difficult if you have dentures or sore gums.

◆ Health issues: Health problems, medications, and over-the-counter drugs can hinder appetite. These changes may be coupled with other age-related complications as in digestive difficulties, oral and dental problems, functional disability, dementia, acute or chronic diseases, and medication-related problems.

During older age your digestive system changes, and you generate less saliva and stomach acid, making it more difficult for your body to process certain vitamins and minerals, such as B12, B6, and folic acid, which are necessary to maintain mental alertness, a keen memory, and good circulation.

◆ Emotional factors: Loneliness and depression can affect your diet. For some, feeling down leads to not eating, while in others it may trigger overeating.

◆ Lifestyle changes: If you live by yourself you may not know how to cook or may not feel like cooking for one.

In addition:

◆ You may need to change your diet to help control conditions such as heart disease, arthritis, and diabetes.

◆ You may be on a restricted diet because of a health condition. Kidney disease is just one example of a condition that often requires restrictions of certain foods or fluids.

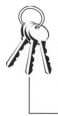

InflamWise

Some older people who have difficulty getting enough daily calories drink nutritional beverages. It is worth noting that a large portion of the calories in these products come from sugar. For example, 201 out of a total of 355 calories in the nutritional drink Ensure come from sugar.

Summing It Up: The Tufts Pyramid

Nutritionists at Tufts University have created specific recommendations for seniors. The recommendations are represented in the pyramid shown. It is particularly geared to help people 50 years or older to eat a healthful diet and put our present-day knowledge about nutrition and aging into action.

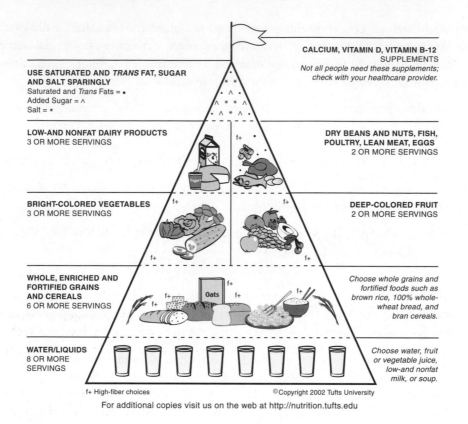

CALCIUM, VITAMIN D, VITAMIN B-12
SUPPLEMENTS
*Not all people need these supplements;
check with your healthcare provider.*

USE SATURATED AND *TRANS* FAT, SUGAR
AND SALT SPARINGLY
Saturated and *Trans* Fats = •
Added Sugar = ∧
Salt = *

LOW-AND NONFAT DAIRY PRODUCTS
3 OR MORE SERVINGS

DRY BEANS AND NUTS, FISH,
POULTRY, LEAN MEAT, EGGS
2 OR MORE SERVINGS

BRIGHT-COLORED VEGETABLES
3 OR MORE SERVINGS

DEEP-COLORED FRUIT
2 OR MORE SERVINGS

WHOLE, ENRICHED AND
FORTIFIED GRAINS
AND CEREALS
6 OR MORE SERVINGS

*Choose whole grains and
fortified foods such as
brown rice, 100% whole-
wheat bread, and
bran cereals.*

WATER/LIQUIDS
8 OR MORE
SERVINGS

*Choose water, fruit
or vegetable juice,
low-and nonfat
milk, or soup.*

f+ High-fiber choices   ©Copyright 2002 Tufts University
For additional copies visit us on the web at http://nutrition.tufts.edu

The Tufts nutritionists based the pyramid on this philosophy:

> We know that older people need fewer calories because they tend to be less
> active and their body composition changes. Yet nutrient needs stay the same or
> even increase, so we need to select foods that provide the most nutrients per
> serving. We also know that as individuals age, they lose the sensation of thirst.

The nutritionists also recommend including physical activity such as walking, climb-
ing stairs, or yard work every day.

The base of the pyramid is eight 8-ounce glasses of fluid a day to prevent constipation
and dehydration.

The pyramid is narrower than a traditional pyramid to show that seniors are less
active and require less food to maintain the same weight.

The pyramid emphasizes specific nutrients, such as antioxidants to defend against free
radical damage associated with aging, vitamin D and calcium to keep bones strong,

and folic acid to retain mental acuity and reduce the incidences of stroke and heart disease. To get these nutrients, the pyramid emphasizes nutrient-dense foods such as darker-colored vegetables and fruits that have higher levels of vitamins. Tufts nutritionists suggest …

◆ Dark, leafy greens such as spinach.

◆ Orange and yellow vegetables such as sweet potatoes and squash.

◆ Colorful fruit such as strawberries and mangos that are more rich in vitamins A and C and in folic acid.

◆ Romaine lettuce rather than iceberg.

◆ Peaches, apricots, or nectarines rather than apples, celery, or cucumbers.

Potatoes are not pictured in the pyramid because they are filling but less nutritious.

The nutritionists also stress adequate fiber intake and recommend whole grain products. Because many seniors have problems with bowel function, they emphasize eating whole oranges and carrots rather than just drinking the juice, eating legumes such as beans and lentils instead of meat at least twice a week, and selecting brown rice rather than white.

The scientists stress the inclusion of high-fiber foods in every meal because diets high in fiber are also associated with lower cholesterol levels and reduced risk of cardiovascular disease and cancer.

The Tufts pyramid suggests using fats, oils, and sweets sparingly. It also stresses that older people should limit their intake of desserts and snacks such as cookies and cake that contribute a lot of calories but have few nutrients.

The nutritionists topped the pyramid with a flag as a reminder that older individuals may not get enough of the vitamins that they require for healthy aging. Therefore, some vitamin supplements may be helpful. And extra calcium and vitamin D supplements may be necessary to prevent bone-thinning. They also emphasize that B12 supplements can help to maintain nerve function and reduce the incidence of dementia. According to the Tufts researchers: "Almost a third of older people develop atrophic gastritis and secrete too little gastric acid and pepsin to absorb vitamin B12 from foods. But they can absorb B12 in the pure form available in supplements." The nutritionists also recommend low-fat dairy products such as milk for older adults as excellent sources of calcium, riboflavin, and potassium.

For protein, the Tufts experts recommend grains, beans, fish, chicken with the skin removed, and lean meat.

Here is a summary of how much calcium, vitamin D, and vitamin B12 is needed each day for adults over 50:

◆ Calcium—1,200 milligrams (mg)

◆ Vitamin D—400 IU for adults 51 to 70 and 600 IU for those over 70. Do not exceed these recommendations.

◆ Vitamin B12—2.4 micrograms (mcg)

Pyramid Recommendations

The following sections contain recommendations for each section of the food pyramid.

Low-Fat and Nonfat Dairy

Eat or drink three or more servings of low- or nonfat dairy products. If you have trouble digesting milk products, try lactose-free dairy products, or add lactase to milk.

Examples of serving size: 1 cup low- or nonfat milk or yogurt; 1½ ounces low-fat cheese

Dry Beans and Nuts, Fish, Poultry, Lean Meat, and Eggs

◆ Eat two or more servings of these protein-rich foods.

◆ Beans are a good source of fiber, protein, and other nutrients.

◆ Choose fish, skinless poultry, lean meat, or eggs.

Examples of serving sizes: 1 to 1½ cup cooked lentils or dry beans, 1½ cup chili, 4 tablespoons peanut butter, 2 to 3 ounces fish, skinless poultry, or lean meat—baked, broiled or grilled; ½ cup canned tuna; one egg or ¼ cup egg substitute

Bright-Colored Vegetables

Eat three or more servings of bright colored vegetables. Look for dark green, red, orange, and/or yellow vegetables for best nutrients.

Examples of serving sizes: 1 cup romaine lettuce, ½ cup winter squash or sweet potato, ¾ cup 100 percent vegetable juice, ½ cup carrots, ½ cup cooked spinach

Deep-Colored Fruit

Eat two or more servings of fresh, frozen, dried, or canned fruit packed in juice. Those with deep colors typically have more nutrients. Choose 100 percent fruit juice. Juices fortified with calcium provide a nondairy calcium source.

Examples of serving sizes: one medium peach or banana, ½ cup berries or sliced melon, ¼ cup dried apricots or raisins, ¾ cup 100 percent orange juice

Whole, Enriched, and Fortified Grains and Cereals

Eat six or more servings of high-fiber, fortified, or whole grains such as brown rice, whole-wheat pasta, and bran cereal.

Examples of serving sizes: ½ cup raisin bran or oatmeal, one slice whole-wheat bread, ½ cup cooked enriched pasta or rice

Water/Liquids

Consume eight 8-ounce glasses of water or beverages such as fruit or vegetable juice, milk, reduced-sodium soup, tea or coffee each day.

Examples of serving sizes: 8 ounces water, 8 ounces reduced-sodium soup, 8 ounces nonfat milk

Recipes

Baked Salmon for Two

Recipe makes 4 servings

2½ cups water	1 tsp. dried rosemary
1 cup brown rice	1 tsp. dried basil
1 lb. salmon filet	1 tsp. of dry mustard
¼ cup orange juice	1 tsp. lemon pepper
1 tsp. dried dill weed	

Preheat oven to 350°F. In a saucepan, bring water to a boil. Add rice and stir. Reduce heat, cover, and simmer for 20 minutes.

In a large pan, add enough water to cover the bottom of the pan. Lay the salmon filet in the pan, pink side up. Place cooked rice around the outside of the fish. Sprinkle the orange juice over the fish and rice.

In a small bowl, combine the dill weed, rosemary, basil, mustard, and lemon pepper and sprinkle over the fish and rice. Cover with aluminum foil.

Bake 30 to 40 minutes or until the salmon are tender and flaky.

Greek Spinach Risotto (Spanakorizo)

1 large onion finely sliced

4 cloves garlic, crushed

¼ cup extra-virgin olive oil

1¼ cup brown rice

½ cup chopped parsley

¼ cup chopped oregano

1 large bunch of spinach, washed and chopped

1¼ cup low-fat chicken broth

Juice of ½ a lemon

¼ cup Parmesan cheese

Sauté onion and garlic in olive oil on low heat. Add rice and stir for about 5 minutes till rice is coated with oil (this will stop the rice from sticking together). Add parsley and oregano. Add chopped spinach and stir through.

Place lid on saucepan for a few minutes for spinach to wilt. Add broth and lemon juice and stir to keep the rice from sticking to the bottom of the pot. Simmer for about 15 minutes (rice should still feel a little firm). Turn heat off and let stand till all liquid is absorbed and rice is soft. Serve with Parmesan cheese.

Baked Vegetable Medley with Dill

20 small whole mushrooms (button type keep their shape better than large mushrooms)

1 large bell pepper (red or green), sliced into thin strips

2 zucchinis, sliced

1 carrot, sliced

½ large sweet potato, sliced

1 large red onion, sliced into strips

3 garlic cloves, crushed

⅓ cup extra-virgin olive oil

2 stock cubes dissolved in 1 TB. hot water

2 TB. juice from ½ a lemon

Salt

Place sliced vegetables into a large baking dish. In a small bowl mix olive oil, stock cubes dissolved in water, dill, garlic, lemon. Pour contents of bowl over vegetable mixture and mix through with hands. Cook in preheated oven at 350°F for about 90 minutes or until vegetables are cooked (semi-soft). Drain vegetables and serve.

Healthy (No Lard) Refritos (Refried Beans)

2 cups dried pinto beans, soaked

3 TB. olive oil

2 cups minced onion

6 medium cloves garlic

1½ tsp. salt

Black pepper

Heal olive oil in a skillet. Add 1 cup of onion, 3 cloves of garlic, cumin, and salt. Sauté over medium heat until onions are soft (about 10 minutes). Add the rest of the garlic and add pepper.

Turn heat down and add beans. Mix well. Mash and stir beans with mixture as they soften. Cook until tender.

Gypsy Soup

4 TB. olive oil

2 cups chopped onion

½ cup chopped celery

2 cloves garlic, crushed

2 cups diced peeled sweet potatoes

2 tsp. paprika

1 tsp. ground turmeric

1 tsp. dried basil

1 tsp. salt

1 pinch ground cinnamon

1 pinch cayenne pepper

1 bay leaf

3 cups chicken stock

1 TB. tamari

1 cup chopped fresh tomato

1½ cups cooked garbanzo beans

¾ cup chopped green bell pepper

Heat olive oil in a stockpot over medium-high heat. Sauté onion, garlic, celery and sweet potatoes for about 5 minutes, or until onion is soft. Season with paprika, turmeric, basil, salt, cinnamon, cayenne, and bay leaf. Stir to blend, then stir in chicken stock and tamari. Cover and simmer over low heat for 15 minutes.

Add tomatoes, garbanzo beans, and green pepper to the soup, and simmer for another 10 minutes, or until all of the vegetables are tender. Adjust salt and pepper to taste.

The Least You Need to Know

◆ Stay within a healthy calorie range for your age group.

◆ All seniors should eat plenty of nutrient-dense foods.

◆ People of all ages should drink plenty of water.

Part 3

Anti-Inflammation Guidelines for the Marketplace

Choices! Choices! Choices! With too many choices in restaurants, grocery stores, and at the health-food store, it can be a puzzle to try to pick the foods and supplements that can truly help you beat inflammation. This part of the book covers all the angles, including avoiding the perils at fast-food places, decoding the information on nutrition labels, and the low-down on nutrition supplements.

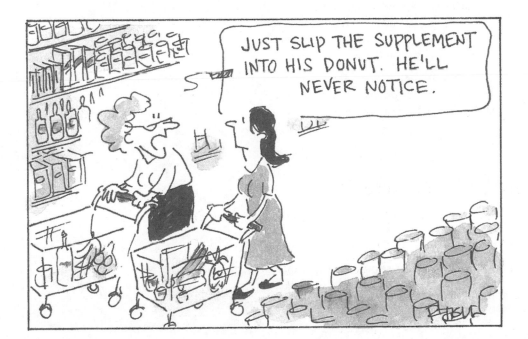

Chapter 13

Fast-Food Survival

In This Chapter

◆ Discover the dangers of fast food, fast-casual food, and restaurant food

◆ Learn tips on eating out and staying on the anti-inflammation diet

◆ Try alternative recipes, including glorious one-pot meals

You know them by their golden arches, "have-it-your-way" slogans, and drive-thru windows—fast-food restaurants are everywhere. In fact, there are now an estimated 250,000 of them in the United States. They dominate our communities. They are even in cafeterias in public schools and hospitals.

In the past, we may have tried to ignore the lack of nutrition in fast food, but we are now becoming aware of just how dangerous fast food is. In recent years the fast food industry has gotten bad press due to the documentary *Super Size Me*, and an increasing awareness of the unhealthiness of the fast food, its key role in the obesity epidemic, and heavy advertising to children. In fact, the publicity has been so bad that the fast-food industry has been trying to change the name of their members to "quick-service restaurants"—with little success.

This chapter covers the dangers and risks of eating fast food in particular and restaurant food in general. We also provide some tips on how to stay on track with the anti-inflammation diet and still drop in at a fast-food counter every once in a while.

Fast Food and the Anti-Inflammation Diet

For a relatively affordable price, fast-food restaurants hand food over to us quickly after we order. Many of us like that convenience, as well as the taste. (Who hasn't ever had a Mac attack?) Many of us go there because our children or grandchildren clamor for "happy meals."

In the United States, most fast-food restaurants belong to a chain or franchise operation. The food they serve (or, more correctly, hand over) is standard from location to location and shipped from headquarters. So is the packaging. The food is highly processed and prepared with a standard formula dictated by headquarters. One of the reliable features of fast-food restaurants is that the products are identical in all respects—from taste to size to packaging. A Whopper is a Whopper wherever you order it.

Fast food has received a super-size chunk of the blame for the obesity epidemic that swept the United States some time ago. It is particularly to blame for the high rate of obesity among children. Its high-fat/empty-calories/low-nutrient fare is responsible for the big waists, metabolic syndrome, and silent inflammation victimizing many a fast-food frequenter.

A Little Background

A White Castle hamburger stand is credited with starting the fast-food craze in 1921. McDonald's, the brand that would become famous for fast food, came on the scene in 1948. Their specialty was hot dogs. Wendy's, founded in 1972, pioneered the drive-thru concept.

In the United States alone, consumers spent about $142 billion on fast food in 2006. But fast food has been losing market share to fast-casual restaurants, which offer somewhat better and more expensive foods. Fast-casual restaurants are similar to fast-food restaurants in that they don't offer full table service. However, they do provide a somewhat higher quality of food and atmosphere and more health-promoting choices. Examples are Boston Market, Noodles and Company, and Panera Bread Co. The typical cost per meal is in the $6 to $10 range. (More on fast-casual restaurants later.)

What the Experts Say

Over the last three decades, fast food has infiltrated every nook and cranny of American society ... Fast food is now served at restaurants and drive-thrus, at stadiums, airports, zoos, high schools, elementary schools, and universities, on cruise ships, trains, and airplanes, at K-Marts, Wal-Marts, gas stations, and even at hospital cafeterias.

In 1970, Americans spent about $6 billion on fast food; in 2000, they spent more than $110 billion. Americans now spend more money on fast food than on higher education, personal computers, computer software, or new cars. They spend more on fast food than on movies, books, magazines, newspapers, videos, and recorded music combined.

—Eric Schlosser, author of *Fast Food Nation*, HarperPerennial, 2002

Fast Fat

The methods used to cook fast food are part of the reason they are so bad for us. Even though some fast-food restaurants have cleaned up their act and have at least eliminated some trans fats, deep-fried items are still full of bad-for-us fat. As a general rule, fast food is ...

◆ high in bad fats.

◆ high in calories.

◆ high in sodium.

◆ low in fiber.

◆ low in nutrients such as vitamin A, C, D, and folic acid. (The only nutrient that you will get plenty of at a fast-food restaurant is protein, which most of us get too much of anyway.)

What the Experts Say

See, now's the time of the meal when you start getting the McStomachache. You start getting the McTummy. You get the McGurgles in there. You get the McBrick, then you get the McStomachache.

—Morgan Spurlock, while consuming a double quarter-pounder supersize meal for his documentary, *Super Size Me,* in 2004.

Consider these fast-food classics. Remember, the average person needs about 2,000 calories, 65 grams of fat, and no more than 2,400 milligrams of sodium a day.

McDonald's Quarter Pounder with Cheese
530 calories
0 g fiber
30 g fat
51 percent calories from fat
1,310 mg sodium

McDonald's Chicken McNuggets
760 calories
0 g fiber
44 g fat
52 percent calories from fat
1,440 mg sodium

Burger King Whopper with Cheese
780 calories
0 g fiber
47 g fat
54 percent calories from fat
1,390 mg sodium

Burger King BK Broiler (Chicken Sandwich)
550 calories
3 g fiber
25 g fat
46 percent calories from fat
1,110 mg sodium

Kentucky Fried Chicken Original Recipe Chicken—Breast
400 calories
1 g fiber
24 g fat
54 percent calories from fat
1,116 mg sodium

Watch the Fast Fats

Here are some facts on the worst offenders at the fast-food counter.

◆ Fries. One small order of fries has 3 grams of trans fats. The recommendation for trans fats is to eat no more than 2 grams a day (based on a diet of 2,000 calories a day).

◆ Fried chicken and fish. It is difficult to detect just how much trans fat is in these foods because they differ from restaurant to restaurant and item to item. For example, McDonald's Filet-O-Fish has about 1 gram of trans fats while Burger King's Tender Crisp Chicken Sandwich has 4 grams of trans. The smartest approach is to skip anything fried!

◆ Super-sizes (or whatever they are calling it at the time). Unless you are sharing it with a table of eight, skip these items. For example, Hardee's Monster Thickburger has 1,400 calories and 107 grams of fat.

◆ Mayonnaise and other high-fat condiments. Skip the mayo. For example, Burger King's Veggie Burger with regular mayonnaise has 390 calories and 13 grams of fat. Skip the mayo and the veggie burger drops to 310 calories and 7 grams of fat.

◆ Cheese. The cheese on burgers at fast-food restaurants is highly processed. For example, the Burger King Whopper with Cheese has 790 calories and 48 grams of fat. Skip the cheese and the damage drops to 678 calories and 37 grams of fat.

◆ Value Meals. At McDonald's, the medium Extra Value Meal Chicken McGrill supplies half a day's harmful fat and sodium.

Can Fast Equal Nutritious?

With some ingenuity and planning, it is possible to eat fast food every once in a while and cut your nutritional losses. For example, many fast-food chains now disclose trans fats in addition to calories, carbohydrates, salt, and more. However, it is almost impossible to control sodium. Fast food is loaded with it.

Here are some tips for ordering from fast-food restaurants:

Breakfast:

◆ Low-fat whole-grain muffin

◆ Whole-grain bagel with a small amount of light cream cheese, peanut butter, or reduced-fat cheese

- Poached egg or plain scrambled eggs or omelet

- Egg white or egg substitute scrambled eggs or omelet

- Unbuttered whole-grain toast

- Fruit and yogurt

- Oatmeal with non- or low-fat milk

The sandwich counter:

- Sandwich with whole-grain bread

- Lean meat such as ham, chicken, or turkey (no high-fat meats such as bologna or tuna salad!)

- Mustard, or a little ketchup, no mayonnaise

- Lots of tomatoes, lettuce, peppers, and onions

- Green salad, fruit salad, or bean salad

- Unsweetened fruit juice, lower-fat milk, or good old water

The pizza parlor:

- Whole-wheat or other type of whole-grain crust (the thinner, the better)

- Low-fat toppings such as chicken, lean ham, peppers, onion, mushrooms, tomatoes, zucchini, eggplant, or artichokes, reduced-fat cheese

- Vegetarian or Hawaiian pizza

- Light or very little cheese

The Chinese or other Asian stop:

- Barbecued, baked, grilled, or stir-fried chicken, with the skin removed, or seafood

- Grilled chicken sandwich or fajita

- Fresh rice rolls

- Chicken wraps

- Steamed vegetables

- Sushi

- Steamed rice

- Light soy sauce and no MSG

- When ordering stir-fry, be sure to ask for "light" on the fat

The Mexican stop:

- Bean burritos, soft tacos, fajitas, and other nonfried items

- Chicken rather than beef

- Limit refried beans; ask if they have beans that aren't refried

- Pile on extra lettuce, tomatoes, and salsa

- Go easy on cheese, sour cream, and guacamole

- Stay clear of deep-fried taco salad shells; a taco salad can have more than 1,000 calories

The burger stop:

- Children's-size burger with whole-grain bun, no cheese

- Green salad with lower-fat dressing on the side

- Grilled chicken sandwich on whole-grain bun

- Light items

- Skip the mayonnaise or "special sauce"

At the coffee shop:

- Coffee with low-fat milk, café latté or cappuccino made with lower-fat milk

What to Avoid at Fast-Food Restaurants

Here is a quick list of the items you should stay away from at fast-food restaurants:

- Large portions—stick to children's or small sizes

- Chicken nuggets

- Croissant breakfast sandwiches (and croissants or pastries in general)
- Breakfast sandwiches
- Fried fish
- Fried chicken
- Fries
- Onion rings
- Mayonnaise or special sauce

Condiments

Stay away from these unhealthy condiments:

- Butter
- Margarine
- Mayonnaise
- Cheese sauce
- Most "special sauces"

- Tartar sauce
- Sour cream
- Gravy
- Guacamole if made with mayonnaise

The FDA Labeling Law

The Food and Drug Administration sets rules for the claims that can be made in restaurant menus for the nutritional values of individual foods and meals.

Their present rules for restaurants are weak compared to the requirements for foods sold in grocery stores. If a restaurant makes a claim such as "low fat" or "heart healthy" on a menu, the restaurant owner must be able to demonstrate that there is a reasonable basis for believing that the food qualifies to bear this claim.

However, the rules allow restaurants a lot of flexibility in establishing this reasonable basis and in presenting the information to consumers. And their rules affect only those restaurants that place claims such as "low fat" or "heart healthy" on their menus.

> **Did You Know?**
>
> According to the Center for Science in the Public Interest, Americans get about 10 percent of their total calories from fast food.

Unlike processed foods, restaurant menu selections are not required to supply complete nutrition information. In addition, menu items bearing such a claim are not held to the same strict standards of laboratory analyses.

Restaurants can use other more economical methods to meet the standard. For example, a restaurant could show that an item was designed to meet the requirements for the claim because it was prepared using a recipe from a recognized health professional association or dietary group, or that the nutritional values for the dish were calculated using a reliable nutrition database.

Under the rules, nutrition information can be provided to the consumer by any reasonable means. It does not have to be presented in the "Nutrition Facts" format seen on packaged food labels, nor does it have to appear on the menu. For example, a restaurant may compile, in a notebook, information on the fat content of all menu items that bear fat claims so long as the nutrition information is available to consumers upon request.

Casual Fat

The relatively new fast-casual trend in restaurants touts "fresh and healthy ingredients." Examples of these restaurants are Panera, Boston Market, and Baja Fresh. With the impression of made-to-order food and slightly better atmosphere, they have given the fast-food industry a run for its money. But proceed with caution: a lot of the highly appealing food they serve is high in fat and calories (not to mention salt).

Scientists at Tufts' Friedman School of Nutrition, Science, and Policy found that the fat and calorie contents of many of the "healthy" food options at fast-casual restaurants were actually worse than fast food. For example, a Panera Asiago Roast Beef Signature Sandwich (without the chips) has 960 calories and 52 grams of fat. (Compare that to a Big Mac's 570 calories and 34 grams of fat.) Even Panera's Chicken Olivada, which sounds more nutritious, has 750 calories and 28 grams of fat.

 InflamWarnings

You should put salads on your watch list at fast casual restaurants; they are not always as health-promoting as you might wish. A charbroiled chicken salad at Baja Fresh has 590 calories and 22 grams of fat. Replace the chicken with steak and you've signed on to pack in 700 calories and 31 grams of fat. And Boston Market's Caesar salad has 140 calories and 8 grams of fat. Not too bad, right? A serving of salad dressing adds an additional 360 calories and 38 grams of fat.

Most breads and bakery products in fast-casual restaurants come with a touch of culture. (They have names like "Ciabatta" and "Artisan Three Seed.") But they are made with refined flour. Soups are also often high in calories and fat. An 8-ounce serving of Panera's broccoli cheddar soup has 230 calories and 16 grams of fat. And 6 ounces of Boston Market's Chicken Tortilla soup with toppings has 350 calories and 21 grams of fat. It is also loaded with trans fats!

Cold and Sweet Fats

If you think ice cream is a necessary part of life, you are in good company. The French philosopher Voltaire said, "Ice cream is exquisite. What a pity it isn't illegal." To many of us, ice cream is necessary for peace of mind. But to remind you of how much that double dip might cost you, here are some facts. Keep in mind that the fat in ice cream is mostly a bad-for-you fat.

◆ Ben and Jerry's Cherry Garcia Original Ice Cream, ½ cup: 260 calories and 14 grams of fat.

◆ Cold Stone Creamery's Black Cherry, 6 ounces: 394 calories and 22 grams of fat

But, here are some lower-damage alternatives:

◆ Cold Stone Creamery Sweet Cream—Nonfat, 6 ounces: 220 calories, no fat

◆ Ben and Jerry's Cherry Garcia Frozen Yogurt, ½ cup: 170 calories and 3 grams of fat.

Fast Fat and Kids

Here's a startling fact: nearly one third of children eat fast food every day, according to a Harvard study reported in the journal *Pediatrics*. The study looked at over 6,000 kids. Those who ate fast food took in, on average, 187 calories more each day than the kids who did not. They also consumed an average of 9 grams more fat, 24 grams more carbs, 26 grams more sugar, and 228 grams more sweetened drinks. The differences add up to about 6 pounds of extra weight per year in the average child who eats fast food—from eating fast food two or three times a week. They eat fewer fruits and vegetables, drink less milk, and get less fiber.

There is no doubt love for fast food has contributed to the surge in obesity among children in the United States. As we mention in Chapter 12, obesity in kids has reached epidemic levels. Experts estimate that 15 percent of kids are overweight and another 15 percent are high risk of becoming overweight. And two thirds of these overweight kids will become overweight adults.

Here are some tips about fast food and kids:

◆ Soda is high in empty calories and it provides no nutrition. See if you can substitute water or milk.

◆ Kids love chicken nuggets. A kid's portion (four pieces) of Wendy's Chicken Nuggets has 200 calories and 14 grams of fat, 2 of which are trans fats! Try to steer them away.

◆ Skip the fries, try taking along a bag of cut up vegetables and fruit instead. This will add vitamins and fiber to the meal. In addition, a lot of places are now offering fruit instead of fries.

Sit-Down Fat

Restaurants that are slower and have wait staffs, sit-down tables, nonplastic silverware, and food that is reportedly cooked to order are not required to tell you what fats they cook with or anything else about the ingredients in your food. (Well, fast- and casual-food restaurants don't have to either, but public pressure has resulted in more and more restaurants revealing their ingredients.)

When eating out, it is important to think in terms of not going off of your anti-inflammation diet, but that dining is part of it. Order wisely. If portions are big and/or the food is high in fat and empty calories, try to share it or leave some on your plate. Don't take it home! That just extends the harm to the next day.

Here are some tips to help keep you on the anti-inflammation diet while dining out.

◆ Some restaurants will meet your special needs if you phone ahead. Ask if your food can be prepared with olive oil, little salt, no butter, no fatty sauce, and broiled instead of fried.

◆ Try to avoid buffets. All-you-can-eat seems like a good deal, but buffets promote eating too much. It is hard to resist that chocolate cream pie when you have already paid for it!

◆ Consider snacking on a health-promoting, filling snack before you go out to eat. This is also a great way to keep from eating or drinking too much at parties. Here is what can happen: when you arrive at a restaurant or party feeling hungry, you may launch into the first offering of food, which is often the bread basket, heavy appetizers, and salty snacks.

◆ When you first sit down, ask your server not to bring the bread basket or chips. It's easier to avoid temptation if you don't even have to look at the bait.

◆ Many restaurants now offer healthy choices on their menus, and the good sit-down restaurants will modify menu items on your request. If not, consider going some-where else. Many restaurants also provide nutritional information on all of their offerings if you ask for it. A simple, "Does this come without the cream sauce?" or "Can you grill that with olive oil instead of butter?" could keep you on track.

◆ If you don't know what's in a dish or don't know the serving size, ask.

◆ Main courses that have been baked, broiled, roasted, poached, or steamed are more health promoting than anything fried.

◆ Salads with plenty of fresh fruits and vegetables and lighter dressings are better than salads with croutons, cheeses, meats, and heavy dressings.

◆ Most restaurants have foods that fit with the anti-inflammation diet, but they are served in butter and heavy sauces. Request that your entrées and sides be served without them.

◆ Ask if it is possible to order a smaller portion (often called "half sizes"), that will help eliminate the temptation to overeat.

◆ If you are on a low-salt meal plan, ask that no salt be added to your food.

◆ Sharing entrées, appetizers, and desserts with dining partners is a great idea.

◆ Order salad dressing on the side, so that you can control the amount that you eat. Vinegar and a dash of oil or a squeeze of lemon are a better choice than high-fat dressings.

If you like the cooperation and choices you have at a particular restaurant, let the manager and chef know. If you want more health-promoting choices, also let them know.

Health-promoting choices at sit-down restaurants:

◆ Appetizers: tomato juice; soup (not cream based); consommé; raw vegetables such as celery or radishes (skip the dip); fresh fruit; fresh, steamed seafood, no mayonnaise

◆ Eggs: poached, boiled; egg whites; egg replacements

◆ Salads: tossed vegetable; spinach; sliced tomato; cucumber; low-fat cottage cheese; low-fat dressing, lemon juice, vinegar, or a splash of oil and vinegar

◆ Entrées: fish, lean meat with the skin removed, vegetarian choices if they are made without bad fats

◆ Breads: anything whole-grain, skip the crackers

◆ Starches: skip potatoes and white rice, request whole grains like wild rice

◆ Vegetables: raw, stewed, steamed, or boiled

◆ Desserts: fresh fruit, fat-free or low-fat yogurt, low-fat ice cream, frozen yogurt or sorbet

Sit-Down Restaurant Tips

Stay away from anything with these labels:

Alfredo	Crispy	Rich sauce
Allemande sauce	Deep-fried	Sautéed
Au gratin	En croûte	Scalloped
Cheese sauce	Fried	Supreme sauce
Battered	Hollandaise	Thai peanut sauce (or any sauce made with coconut milk)
Béchamel	Horseradish sauce (plain horseradish is fine)	
Béarnaise sauce		Veloute sauce
Breaded	Newburg sauce	White sauce
Buttered	Pan-fried	With gravy
Butter sauce	Pastry	With thick sauce
Creamed	Remoulade	

And stay away from foods high in salt:

Pickled

Smoked

Soy sauce

A Note About Slow Food

Slow food is a movement formed as an international backlash to fast food. The founding father of the Slow Food Movement, Carlo Petrini, recognized in 1986 that the "industrialization of food" was leading to the destruction of thousands of "natural" food varieties and flavors.

Concerned that the world was quickly reaching a point of no return, he wanted to reach out to consumers and demonstrate to them that they have choices over fast food and supermarket homogenization. He rallied his friends and began to speak out at every available opportunity, and soon the Slow Food Movement was born. Today the organization is active in 50 countries and has a worldwide membership of over 80,000.

Slow Food U.S.A. supports and celebrates the food traditions of North America. Some of its goals include promoting pure food that is local, seasonal, and organically grown—a goal that fits nicely with the anti-inflammation approach to diet and lifestyle.

Breakfast Recipes and Tips

The following sections provide some ideas for replacing fast fats and other offending restaurant foods for breakfast.

Fresh Fruit Salad

Mix together bite-size pieces of your favorite fruits, such as pineapple, mango, banana, berries, or apple. Toss them with some fresh mint, cinnamon, or ginger. Top with low-fat yogurt. You can make the salad the night before you eat it. Be sure to coat apples and other fruit with lemon or orange juice to prevent browning.

Hot Cereal

Sprinkle your hot amaranth or oatmeal with chopped prunes, walnuts, and applesauce. Oat-based cereals have a low glycemic index, which means they are gradually absorbed and digested by the body. (But they do have gluten, if this is an issue for you.)

Frozen Berries

Keep frozen berries in the freezer, and defrost the night before you want to use them. You can use them in yogurt, sprinkled on muesli, or in smoothies. Sweeten to taste.

Breakfast Drinks

If you prefer to drink your breakfast, try making a smoothie at home, such as this recipe. Put everything into the blender the night before and store in the fridge.

Basic Smoothie

½ cup nonfat milk

½ cup fat-free plain yogurt

½ frozen banana, peeled and chopped

2 TB. powdered protein supplement

1½ TB. flaxseed

1 tsp. honey

½ cup frozen strawberries, blueberries, or other fruit

In a blender, blend the milk, yogurt, banana, protein supplement, flaxseed, honey, and strawberries until smooth.

Stay Away from Store-Bought Breakfast Bars

Breakfast bars are composed mostly of sugar and other carbohydrates. For example, Starbucks' Apricot Granola Bar has 470 calories, 25 grams of fat, and 56 grams of carbohydrate. Contrary to what you would expect, it also has no vitamin C. Its only real nutritive value is vitamin A. This is typical of most breakfast bars, although they may advertise lower calories, which is true only because they are smaller in size.

Apricot Squares

1½ cups chopped dried apricots

2 cups water

¼ cup raw honey

1½ cups oat flakes

1½ cups whole-wheat flour

½ cup chopped walnuts

½ cup unrefined or cold-pressed oil

½ cup raw honey

Mix apricots, water, and ¼ cup honey in saucepan. Bring to boil and then simmer uncovered on low heat for 10 minutes.

Mix oat flakes, flour, walnuts, oil, and ½ cup honey and press half of mix into bottom of 8×8 pan. Spread apricot mix on top and sprinkle the rest of the oat mix on top. Bake 20 to 30 minutes at 350°F until lightly browned. Cool and cut into 16 squares.

Homemade Breakfast Bars

1 cup whole-grain cereal	½ tsp. salt
¾ cup oats (not instant)	1 tsp. cinnamon
½ cup whole-wheat flour	6 oz. nonfat yogurt
1½ tsp. ground flax seeds	1 large egg
1½ tsp. wheat germ	1 egg white
⅓ cup chopped walnuts	½ cup applesauce or prune purée
¼ cup 70 percent cocoa chocolate chips	⅓ cup sugar
½ tsp. baking soda	

Combine cereal, oats, whole-wheat flour, flaxseeds, wheat germ, nuts, chocolate chips, baking soda, salt, and cinnamon in a large mixing bowl. Add remaining ingredients and stir to combine.

Pour into lightly sprayed 9×9 dish. Bake at 350°F for 20 to 25 minutes.

Fruit and Spice Breakfast Bulgur

2 apples

1½ cups + 2 TB. unsweetened
apple juice

½ tsp. vanilla

¼ tsp. salt

1 TB. grated orange peel

1½ cups bulgur

1½ cups dried cranberries

½ cup unsalted peanuts

Chop the apples into small chunks and sprinkle with 2 tablespoons
apple juice to prevent browning. Place 1½ cups apple juice into
a heavy bottomed sauce pan and add the vanilla, salt, and orange
peel. Bring mixture to a boil. Stir in the bulgur, then cover the pan
and reduce the heat to medium low. Simmer the bulgur for approximately 15 minutes, or until the liquid is absorbed. Mix in apple
chunks, dried cranberries, and peanuts.

Lunch Recipes and Tips

Taking a salad to the office is easy. Put your vegetable mix, spinach, or lettuce in a bag
and put a damp paper towel on top. Take the dressing in a separate jar.

Take homemade soups in thermos flasks, or make your own healthy sandwich.

The following sections provide some ideas for replacing fast fats and other offending
restaurant foods for lunch.

Whole-Grain Vegetable Sandwiches

2 slices whole-grain bread

½ avocado, mashed

1 tomato, sliced

½ small cucumber, sliced

Little Spanish onion, thinly
sliced

Other vegetables of your
choice, such as grated carrots
or sliced beets

2 tsp. canola mayonnaise
(available in health-food
store)

Salt and pepper to taste

Evenly spread the mashed avocado on one slice of the whole-grain bread and lightly sprinkle the salt and pepper over the avocado. Spread mayonnaise on the remaining slice of bread. Add the tomato, cucumber, onion, and other vegetables to make two sandwiches.

Turkey BLT Wrap

1 TB. fat-free mayonnaise

1 flour tortilla

3 slices turkey bacon, cooked

3 oz. roast turkey breast, diced

2 slices tomato

2 leaves lettuce

Smear the mayonnaise on the tortilla. Line the middle of the tortilla with the bacon and top with the turkey breast, tomato, and lettuce. Roll the whole thing tightly into a tube.

Hummus with Yogurt and Lemon

This is an adaptation of Middle Eastern garbanzo bean dip. Yogurt replaces some of the high-fat tahini (sesame seed paste). The dip is great as a lunch with fresh vegetables or toasted whole-grain pita bread wedges.

2 large garlic cloves

1 (15-oz.) can garbanzo beans (chickpeas), drained

2 TB. plain nonfat yogurt

2 TB. tahini

2 TB. fresh lemon juice

1 tsp. ground cumin

Mince garlic in processor. Add remaining ingredients; blend until coarse purée forms, occasionally scraping down sides of work bowl. Season hummus to taste with salt and pepper. Transfer to small bowl. (Can be prepared 3 days ahead. Cover and refrigerate. Bring to room temperature before serving.)

Dinner Recipes and Tips

The following sections provide some ideas for replacing fast fats and other offending restaurant foods for dinner.

Broccoli Soup

Make this soup at home instead of buying the high-fat version from one of the fast-casual restaurants. Serve with a salad with Green Goddess dressing (recipe below).

2 cups nonfat chicken or vegetable broth

4 cups chopped fresh broccoli

1 cups chopped celery

1 cups chopped carrots

½ cup chopped onion

1 tsp. flour

6 TB. olive or canola oil

2 cups low-fat milk

1 TB. minced fresh parsley

1 tsp. onion salt

½ tsp. garlic powder

½ tsp. salt

In a Dutch oven or soup kettle, bring water to a boil. Add broccoli, celery, and carrots; boil 2 to 3 minutes. Drain; set vegetables aside. In the same pan, sauté onion in olive oil until tender. Stir in flour. Gradually add the broth and milk, stirring constantly. Bring to a boil; boil and stir for 1 minute. Add vegetables and remaining ingredients. Reduce heat; cover and simmer 30 to 40 minutes or until vegetables are tender.

Green Goddess Dressing

1 avocado

1½ cup fat-free buttermilk

1 clove garlic

¼ cup chopped cilantro, Italian parsley, or mint

2 TB. rice vinegar

½ tsp. salt

Mix ingredients in a blender. You can also try adding a little canola mayonnaise for a thicker consistency.

More from Elizabeth Yarnell

Try these quick and nutritious recipes from Elizabeth Yarnell. These recipes are fast and delicious, while being the antithesis of fast food.

African Peanut Butter Stew

½ onion, diced

¾ cup brown rice, dry

1¼ cup and 1 TB. water or nonfat broth

2 pieces chicken

½ orange bell pepper

⅔ cup skim milk or water

2–4 cloves garlic, minced and crushed

½ tsp. cayenne pepper

Salt to taste

3 TB. all natural peanut butter, creamy or chunky

3–4 tomatoes, or 1 (14-oz.) can drained

1 carrot, diced

1 handful spinach leaves or 5 frozen

Preheat oven to 450°F. Spray inside of 2-quart Dutch oven and lid with canola oil or wipe with peanut oil.

Place onions, rice, and water or broth in bottom of pot and smooth into an even layer. Rinse chicken and place on rice in single layer. Add bell pepper slices.

In a measuring cup, whisk milk, garlic, cayenne pepper, salt, and peanut butter until you have a thick, soupy paste. Pour over chicken. Layer in tomatoes, carrots, and spinach.

Cover and bake. Check after 45 minutes; you may want to leave it in the oven for another 15 minutes. Notes from Elizabeth Yarnell: If using a can of tomatoes, drain the liquid into a measuring cup, fill with water to make ¾ cup and 1 tablespoon and use to mix with rice.

For fun variations try:

◆ Chicken or vegetable broth instead of milk. You can also substitute soy or rice milk.

◆ Try a minced jalapeño pepper instead of the cayenne. Or use four shakes of red pepperoncini flakes.

◆ Shrimp and/or scallops instead of or along with chicken tastes great, too. Or try firm tofu.

◆ Try sweet potatoes instead of rice.

Stuffed Cabbage Leaves

¼ cup barley

½ cup water

Salt and pepper to taste

1 (14-oz.) can tomatoes

1 lemon squeezed or juiced

1 tsp. sugar (optional)

1 egg, lightly beaten

½ onion, peeled and chopped

1 carrot, washed, grated or minced

¼ lb. lean ground turkey

1 TB. parsley, minced (optional)

1–3 cloves garlic, peeled and minced

6–8 leaves white cabbage, washed, intact

Preheat oven to 450°F. Spray inside of 2-quart Dutch oven and lid with canola oil or wipe with peanut oil.

Pour barley in a strainer and rinse in cold water. In a small bowl, mix barley with ½ cup water, lightly salt and pepper and set aside. Drain tomatoes and reserve the strained liquid. Squeeze lemon into tomato liquid, add sugar if desired, and lightly salt and pepper.

Gently beat egg in medium mixing bowl. Add in onions, carrots, turkey, parsley, and garlic. Add tomatoes. Lightly salt and pepper. Blend well with a fork.

Pour barley mixture into pot and spread into even layer. Place a row of cabbage leaves on top of water level. Scoop half of ground meat mixture in and drench with half tomato juice mixture. Add a layer of cabbage leaves and rest of turkey mixture. Cover with rest of the leaves and finish with rest of the tomato juice mixture.

Cover and bake for 45 to 50 minutes or until the aroma fills the kitchen (about 3 minutes past first sniff).

Teriyaki Tempeh

1 cup brown rice

1¼ cup plus 1 tsp. water

1 (8-oz.) package tempeh, cut into strips

1 tsp. Chinese five-spice powder

1 TB. low-sodium soy sauce

1 TB. hoisen sauce

1 TB. peanuts, crushed or peanut oil

¼ head cabbage, purple, shredded

2 carrots, sliced in thin ovals

1 (8-oz.) can water chestnuts, sliced

Preheat oven to 450°F. Spray inside of 2-quart Dutch oven and lid with canola oil or wipe with peanut oil.

Rinse rice in strainer under cold water until water runs clear and place in bottom of pot. Add water and spread into thin layer. Dust tempeh strips with five-spice powder and set in pot.

In a small bowl, mix together soy sauce, hoisen sauce, and peanuts or peanut oil to make teriyaki sauce. Spoon half mixture over tempeh. Add thick layer of cabbage and continue to add carrots, mushrooms, and water chestnuts. Pour rest of sauce over all.

Cover and bake for 45 minutes.

Notes from Elizabeth Yarnell:

◆ Feel free to substitute 3 tablespoons prepared teriyaki sauce for the soy/hoisen/peanut mixture.

◆ Almost any vegetable tastes stupendous teriyaki-style. Try this recipe with broccoli, cauliflower, Brussels sprouts, spinach, bell peppers, zucchini, or any other vegetable you happen to have available.

Greek Chicken

½ cup whole-wheat couscous, dry

½ cup + 1 TB. water or fat-free broth

2–3 skinned chicken thighs or breasts

Salt and pepper to taste

4–7 cloves garlic

1 TB. capers, drained

2 TB. parsley, chopped

1 cup Kalamata olives, pitted, halved

1 small zucchini, medallions

3 tomatoes, sliced

Preheat oven to 450°F. Spray inside of 2-quart Dutch oven and lid with canola oil or wipe with peanut oil.

Spread raw, dry couscous in an even layer in bottom of the pot. Add water or broth and swirl to coat all the grains and spread them evenly. Place rinsed chicken pieces in a single layer (it is okay if they are slightly submerged). Season the chicken with salt and pepper, then sprinkle with garlic, capers, and half the parsley.

Add the olives, zucchini, and tomatoes. Sprinkle with the rest of the parsley and lightly season with salt and pepper.

Cover and bake for 45 minutes.

Notes from Elizabeth Yarnell: Substitute an 8-ounce can of ripe pitted California olives for Kalamata, a 15-ounce can of diced tomatoes for fresh tomatoes, and 1½ cups of frozen broccoli florets for the zucchini to change this meal from a taste of summer to an easy mid-winter dish.

The Least You Need to Know

◆ Fast food is fast fat.

◆ Fast food is partly responsible for the obesity epidemic among children.

◆ It is possible to eat in a fast-food, fast-casual, or sit-down restaurant and stay on the anti-inflammation diet; however, you need to make wise choices.

Chapter 14

Food Shopping Strategies

In This Chapter

◆ Guidelines for shopping in grocery stores

◆ How to organize your anti-inflammation shopping list

◆ How to read ingredient labels

◆ Understanding genetically modified foods

◆ How to use certification programs to guarantee quality

There are good reasons why grocery shopping can be daunting. In fact, there are tens of thousands of reasons. The average store has over 30,000 items. And the items vary from store to store.

Going to the grocery store and trying to understand the small print on thousands of food labels can be overwhelming. However, determining whether a particular product fits into the anti-inflammation diet is important. To guarantee that you are getting wholesome foods with your grocery dollars, this chapter provides a simplified guide to shopping for food and reading food labels. It also includes genetically modified foods and reducing contamination from packaged foods.

Food Shopping Savvy

The following sections include guidelines to follow when you shop in a grocery store.

Although some of the choices in these sections are low in bad fats and high in health-promoting foods, they may be hidden among refined and processed foods, or foods high in harmful fats. As always, make sure you read labels carefully.

The Produce Section

Learn to love the produce section. Fill your cart about two thirds with fruits and vegetables. Find enough produce to equal nine servings a day (see Chapter 10). Make choices from at least three different colors.

The Fish Counter

Your best friend is the person who stocks the fish counter. Shop for fatty fish that are high in omega-3s: turbot, salmon, herring, mackerel, sardines, Atlantic bluefish, most shellfish, Pacific oysters, squid, and anchovies. Stay way from anything breaded—fresh or frozen. Don't buy the tarter sauce displayed on top of the sneeze guard. It is basically high-fat mayonnaise with some relish thrown in.

Uncooked Beans and Whole Grains

Branch out and try some whole grains and legumes that you have not eaten before such as amaranth or red lentils. If you buy pasta, go for whole grain.

Dry beans are the best deal in town. You can make a black-bean soup that serves six for pennies. Serve it with whole-grain rice for nutritional clout. And don't forget the flax!

The Dairy Section

Choose fat-free and low-fat products over the high-fat options. Go for low-fat or nonfat milk, yogurt, and cottage cheese. Stay away from the butter and margarines. You may want to try one of the spreads with plant sterols such as Benacol.

Look for these items in the dairy section:

- 1 percent milk
- Skim milk

- Nonfat yogurt—sugar-free
- Low-fat varieties of cheese
- Buttermilk
- Nonfat dry milk
- Evaporated skim milk

- Reduced or nonfat cream cheese
- Farmer's cheese
- Reduced or fat-free sour cream
- Low or nonfat cottage cheese

InflamWise

If you can't stand the taste of a low-fat version of a product, try another option with slightly more fat. Sometimes just a touch of fat can make a lot of difference in taste and not break your fat bank. For example, if you don't like nonfat cottage cheese, try the 1 percent version to see if that appeals more. It is still a big improvement over eating the full-fat version.

Eggs

Eggs are a great source of protein, iron, and other nutrients, but are high in cholesterol. And the yolk of one egg has 5 grams of fat. Purchasing just the white of eggs is a great option. Egg substitutes are generally also a great choice.

InflamWise

Not all eggs are alike. Some producers feed their hens all-vegetarian feed that contains no animal fat, no animal by-products, and no recycled or processed food. The result is eggs that are lower in cholesterol and saturated fat and higher in omega-3 fatty acids than conventional eggs. Examples of producers to check out are Eggland's Best Eggs, Egg Innovations, and Organic Valley.

The Freezer

Walk right past the ice cream section. (If you purchase a low-fat or fat-free frozen dairy product, choose a small size. A serving, which may still have a couple of hundred calories, is half a cup—less than a normal scoop.) Also skip the frozen convenience foods such as pizzas and sandwich pockets.

Proceed to the frozen vegetables and fruits. Read every label carefully, and be on the lookout for additives. Stay away from vegetables in sauces.

The Bakery

Walk past the donuts and look for whole-grain products such as whole-wheat bread or bagels. Don't be fooled by labels that say "wheat." It means that the product is made from a mixture of white and whole-wheat flours. To be labeled whole wheat, the product must say whole wheat.

Here are a couple of other tips:

◆ Buy whole-grain breads that say they have at least 2 grams of fiber per slice.

◆ If you want to cut back on calories, buy the thinly sliced whole-wheat bread that has 40 to 60 calories per slice.

The Cereal Aisle

It requires a fair amount of work to find a cereal that is not loaded with sugar. Even most granolas are packed with it—and a large amount of fat. Buy only the cereals that have less than 8 grams of sugar per serving. Examples are Shredded Wheat, the original Cheerios, Wheaties, and Total.

Surprisingly, cereals also contain a lot of salt. Stock up on whole grains such as amaranth and oats to replace ready-made cereals.

The Meat Counter

The rule here is lean—the leaner, the better. If you plan to cook poultry with the skin left on, take it off after cooking and dab with a paper towel before eating.

If you are buying beef, choose lean cuts and trim all visible fat before cooking. Trimming the fat does not reduce the vitamin and mineral quality of the meat.

The top five lean cuts of meat are top round, eye of round, round tip, bottom round, and shank.

Try buffalo—it has a taste similar to beef and is leaner.

The leanest cuts of lamb are leg of lamb, foreshank, lean loin chop, lamb loin chop, and lamb roast.

The leanest cuts of pork are tenderloin, center loin chops, lean ham, sirloin roast, top loin roast, Canadian bacon, rib chops, and shoulder blade steak.

Avoid fatty processed meats, such as bacon and sausage. They not only contain lots of saturated fat but also may contain nitrates. And only a saltlick would contain more sodium.

Proceed with Extreme Caution

The foods in this section are only for special occasions.

Deli Don'ts

Unless labeled low-fat (or reduced fat), assume that all prepared items (salads, slaws, tuna and other seafood mixtures) are being exceptionally high in fat and sodium. Even the fruit salad is often off limits. It may have added sugars.

 InflamWarnings

Many people assume that if you purchase your meats at a deli counter it means they are healthier. Not necessarily so. Many contain additives, preservatives, and meat by-products. Ask the clerk behind the counter if you can read the package label of any product you are considering.

Packaged and Convenience Foods

Make these convenience items off limits as much as you can: seasoned rices, convenience soups, and meals in boxes. Many are high in fat and have lots of salt and processed or refined additives.

Most rice mixes contain anywhere from 600 to 1,000 mg of sodium per serving. Some have much more. Rice-A-Roni's Yellow Rice and Rice-Pilaf have close to 1,800 mg per serving! That's close to a teaspoon of salt, and almost as much as the National Academy of Sciences says should be the daily limit. Pre-packaged mixes can also be high in fat. For example, Budget Gourmet's Oriental Rice has 2½ teaspoons of fat in its ½-cup servings.

The Candy Aisle

Stay away as often as you can, particularly if you have kids in your cart. However, chocolate that is more than 70 percent cocoa is actually great for you in small amounts.

> **InflamWise**
>
> Here are some tips to cut down on the salt and fat in packaged mixes:
>
> Buy the brands that have separate seasoning packets and use only half the packet. And if the mix calls for added fat, use only half of the recommended amount or do not add any at all.
>
> Or, for a healthy and yummy alternative, cook brown rice in seasoned (unsalted) stock. When cooked, sauté it with olive oil and a little onion, add a touch of your favorite spice such as curry or chili powder, and serve. This mix is great with chunks of winter squash, pearl onions, and peas. (It's fine to use the frozen varieties.)
>
> Try a similar technique with whole-grain pasta. Cook the pasta, drain, and mix in a pan with olive oil, sautéed onion and garlic, and cooked vegetables of your choice.

The Snack Aisle

Stay away, but see the list later on in this chapter about healthy snacks.

Condiments

Here is a list of the best choices for condiments:

- Ketchup
- Mustard
- Low-sodium soy sauce
- Low-sodium teriyaki sauce
- Balsamic vinegar
- Barbecue sauce
- White wine vinegar
- Cider vinegar
- Lemon juice
- Worcestershire sauce
- Salsa
- Spices such as fines herbs, basil, oregano, garlic, cayenne, and dill

Pantry Items

Here is a list of the best choices to stock up on for your pantry:

- Olive oil
- Canola oil

- Nonstick cooking sprays
- Fat-free and low-fat salad dressings
- Balsamic vinegar
- Low-fat mayonnaise
- Soy mayonnaise

- Canola mayonnaise
- Natural peanut butter
- Almond butter
- Tahini

InflamWise

While both ketchup and barbecue sauce are okay when used in small amounts, be sure to use sparingly. They are very high in sodium and sugar. For example, 1 tablespoon of ketchup has 15 calories and 167 mg of sodium, and 1 tablespoon of barbecue sauce has 20 calories and 208 mg of sodium.

(The National Academy of Sciences recommends that the daily allowance for sodium is 5.8 grams per day.)

Making a Grocery List

A list can keep you on track—especially if you keep your anti-inflammation diet in mind. Professional organizers suggest grouping similar items together on your list. To save time, you might develop a form you can photocopy or print from your computer for weekly use. Keep your list in a central location where your family can add to it as needed.

Remember that time spent developing a list is usually less than time spent returning to the store for a forgotten item.

You may want to make a list for your various shopping destinations such as the grocery store, farmer's market, discount center, and so on.

The Master List

Here are some tips for developing a master list for ongoing use.

- Consider listing foods by categories based on the Healthy Eating Pyramid or, if over age 70, the Tufts Pyramid for People 70+. This will help assure that your meals will fit within the anti-inflammation diet.

◆ Some organizational experts recommend arranging the categories in their list around the order in which foods are stocked in the store you frequent most often. However, stores can change where they place foods.

◆ Make sure to include a catch-all grouping for condiments, staples, and other food items that don't fit anywhere else.

◆ If there are foods and other items that you eat regularly, give yourself a reminder by making them a permanent part of your master list. For example, if you always like to have some carrots in the house, write "carrots" under your Vegetable category heading. Then, if you need carrots that week, circle that item.

Suggested Category Headings

Here are some sample category headings for a master list and an example of one possible must-have item you might include under each. Use these examples as a guideline in creating your own personalized list and must-have weekly foods for your family:

◆ Eggs and dairy

◆ Freezer

◆ Bakery

◆ Cereals

◆ Dairy

◆ Lean meats

◆ Deli items

◆ Condiments

◆ Pantry items

InflamWise _____

For some foods, you may want to wait until you're at the store before deciding what specific items to buy. For example, you may wish to see if strawberries are on sale or which vegetables have come into season. To avoid multiple trips to the grocery store, write on your list the number of things you need from each group. For example, if you need lean protein for seven meals, write "seven lean proteins."

Farmer's Markets and Co-Ops

When possible, visit farmers' markets and produce stands in your area for fresh foods. Food co-ops are another good source of healthy food. These groups tend to buy organic or pesticide-free produce. Health food markets and specialty stores also can be worth the extra trip to find a wider variety of foods and brands.

Nutrition Facts		
Serving Size 1 cup (228g)		
Servings Per Container 2		
Amount Per Serving		
Calories 250	Calories from Fat 110	
		% Daily Value*
Total Fat 12g		18%
Saturated Fat 3g		15%
Trans Fat 3g		
Cholesterol 30 mg		10%
Sodium 470mg		20%
Total Carbohydrate 31g		10%
Dietary Fiber 0g		0%
Sugars 5g		
Protein 5g		
Vitamin A		4%
Vitamin C		2%
Calcium		20%
Iron		4%

* Percent Daily Values are based won a 2,000 calorie diet. Your Daily Values may be higher or lower depending on your calorie needs.

	Calories:	2,000	2,500
Total Fat	Less than	65g	80g
Sat Fat	Less than	20g	25g
Cholesterol	Less than	300mg	300mg
Sodium	Lessthan	2,400mg	2,400mg
Total Carbohydrate		300g	375g
Dietary Fiber		25g	730g

How to Read Nutritional Labels

Food labels are designed to help you make healthy food choices, but they take a little detective work. How do you make sense of them? The following sections provide details on how to decipher food labels.

All packaged food products are required by the Nutrition Labeling and Education Act to contain the following information:

- ◆ Common name of the product
- ◆ Name and address of the product's manufacturer
- ◆ Net contents

Nutrition Facts

Common nutrients, such as total fat, cholesterol, and sodium, are required fields. Other nutrients, such as potassium and vitamin K, are optional and not required to be listed. Each package must identify the quantities of specified nutrients and food constituents for one serving. It is important to note the following:

Food	Number of Calories
1 g of fat	9
1 g of protein	4
1 g of carbohydrate	4
1 g of alcohol	7

Serving Size

Serving sizes are standardized to make for easier comparison among similar food items. They are expressed in both common household and metric measures. It is always important to pay attention to a serving size. For instance, a serving of chocolate chip cookies is typically two pieces. Hence, if you eat four pieces, you will need to double the nutritional information.

This is an area that can easily trip you up. Do you really eat the amount listed on the package as one serving? For example, one bag of Glenny's Soy Crisps contains two servings of crisps. Most of us would polish off the whole bag without thinking. Or what about eating just one serving of ice cream? Or half a can of soup?

Calories (kcal)

Calories provide a measure of how much energy your body gets after eating a portion of food. It is always important to know the total number of calories in a food. Many consumers are surprised to find that a fat-free product is not necessarily low in calories. Similarly, a sugar-free product is not always low in calories or low in fat.

The amount of calories listed on a label refers to the amount in a single serving. If a low-calorie claim appears, the government requires the food distributor to meet these guidelines:

- Calorie-free: Less than 5 calories per serving

- Low-calorie: 40 calories or less, unless it is a main-dish item

- Reduced-calorie: Must have 25 percent less than the regular version

Calories from Fat

The "calories from fat" line provides a measure of how many calories come from fat. Ideally, you want to buy foods with a large gap between total calories per serving and calories from fat. The bigger the gap, the better. For example, let's say that an item such as the macaroni and cheese (see sample) lists 110 calories from fat in one serving. If each serving has a total of 250 calories per serving, then 44 percent of the calories in two servings come from fat (110 divided by 250).

Nutrients Listed

Total fat, saturated fats, cholesterol, total carbohydrate (including fiber and added sugars), protein, vitamins A and C, calcium, and iron are required on the label. Other nutrients are optional and may be listed at the discretion of the manufacturer.

In addition to total calories and total fat, a few other nutrients relevant to heart health are important to pay attention to when reading a label.

Total Fat

This section lists all the total number of fat grams from all types of fats combined.

If a low-fat claim appears, the government requires the food distributor to meet these guidelines:

- Fat-free: less than 0.5 grams of fat

- Low-fat: 3 grams of fat or less

- Reduced fat: At least 25 percent less fat per serving than the original version of the product.

Saturated Fat

This lists how much saturated fat is in the food. You want items that say 0 percent!

Trans Fats

This lists how many trans fatty acids are in the food. You want items that say 0 percent!

Cholesterol

This is the waxy stuff that can clog up your arteries, although it is not as bad for you as saturated fat. The American Heart Association recommends eating less than 200 milligrams of cholesterol per day.

Sodium

General guidelines are 1,200 to 1,300 milligrams per day.

> **InflamWise** _____
>
> As a reminder, salt and sodium are not the same thing. Sodium is an element that joins with chlorine to form sodium chloride, which we know as table salt. Sodium occurs naturally in most foods, but salt is the most common source of sodium in our foods.

Total Carbohydrates

This is the area where you can detect how much of the bad-for-you sugar is in a product. The total carbohydrate line lists how much of all carbohydrates are in a serving of the food. Then, look for the smaller listing, which says "Sugars." This shows how much simple sugar is in a food. You want as little in this line as possible. In other words, the more complex carbohydrates, the better.

Here is an example of how to figure out what proportion of the carbohydrates are complex (relatively good) versus simple (bad). If the total carbohydrate listing reads 15 grams and the simple sugar listing reads 5 grams, then 10 grams are complex. This is not that great because it means a third of this product is composed of simple sugar.

Protein

Most Americans eat way too much protein, and don't have to spend time on this item.

Percent Daily Values

This area assumes that the average person requires 2,000 calories a day. Then, it tells you how much the food supplies for four nutrients—vitamin A, vitamin C, calcium, and iron—and the government's recommendations on how much of that nutrient you should take in. For example, one serving of hearty tomato soup has:

Vitamin A 20%
Vitamin C 40%
Calcium 2%
Iron 6%

This soup is a great source of vitamin C and okay source of vitamin A. It is not a great source for calcium or iron.

Daily Reference Values Footnote

This footnote reminds consumers of the daily intake of different foods depending on their own nutritional needs.

Daily Values for Nutrition

Nutrient	Unit of Measure	Daily Values
Total fat	grams (g)	65
Saturated fatty acids	grams (g)	20
Cholesterol	milligrams (mg)	300
Sodium	milligrams (mg)	2,400
Potassium	milligrams (mg)	3,500
Total carbohydrate	grams (g)	300
Fiber	grams (g)	25
Protein	grams (g)	50
Vitamin A	International Units (IU)	5,000
Vitamin C	milligrams (mg)	60
Calcium	milligrams (mg)	1,000
Iron	milligrams (mg)	18
Vitamin D	International Units (IU)	400

continues

Daily Values for Nutrition   (continued)

Nutrient	Unit of Measure	Daily Values
Vitamin E	International Units (IU)	30
Vitamin K	micrograms (µg)	80
Thiamin	milligrams (mg)	1.5
Riboflavin	milligrams (mg)	1.7
Niacin	milligrams (mg)	20
Folate	micrograms (µg)	400
Vitamin B12	micrograms (µg)	6.0
Biotin	micrograms (µg)	300
Pantothenic acid	milligrams (mg)	10
Phosphorus	milligrams (mg)	1,000
Iodine	milligrams (mg)	400
Zinc	milligrams (mg)	15
Selenium	micrograms (µg)	70
Copper	milligrams (mg)	2.0
Manganese	milligrams (mg)	2.0
Chromium	micrograms (µg)	120
Molybdenum	micrograms (µg)	75
Chloride	milligrams (mg)	3,400

Nutrient Claims—the Basics

What do the various claims on packaged foods mean? What does "natural" mean?

- ◆ Calorie-free: Contains less than 5 calories per serving.

- ◆ Fat-free: Contains less than ½ gram of fat per serving.

- ◆ Fortified: A nutrient that is not naturally present in a food has been added.

- ◆ Good source of fiber: Contains 2.5 to 4.9 grams of fiber per serving.

- ◆ High-fiber: Contains 5 grams of fiber or more per serving. (Foods making high-fiber claims must meet the definition for low-fat, or the level of total fat must appear next to the high-fiber claim.)

♦ Lite: Contains a third of the calories or half the fat per serving of the original version or a similar product.

♦ Low-calorie: Contains a third of the calories of the original version or a similar product.

♦ Low-fat: Contains less than 3 grams of fat per serving. Contains at least 25 percent less per serving than the reference food. (An example might be reduced-fat cream cheese, which would have at least 25 percent less fat than original cream cheese.)

♦ Low-sodium: Contains less than 140 milligrams of sodium per serving.

♦ Lower fat: Contains at least 25 percent less per serving than the reference food. (An example might be reduced-fat cream cheese, which would have at least 25 percent less fat than original cream cheese.)

♦ More or added fiber: Contains at least 2.5 grams more per serving than the reference food.

♦ No calories: Contains less than 5 calories per serving.

♦ No fat: Contains less than ½ gram of fat per serving.

♦ No preservatives added: Contains no added chemicals to preserve the product. Some of these products may contain natural preservatives.

♦ No preservatives: Contains no preservatives (chemical or natural).

♦ No salt or salt-free: Contains less than 5 milligrams of sodium per serving.

♦ Reduced-sugar: Contains at least 25 percent less sugar per serving than the reference food.

♦ Salt-free: Contains less than 5 milligrams of sodium per serving.

♦ Sugar-free: Contains less than ½ gram of sugar per serving.

Remember, these claims are meant to serve as guidelines only.

If you are concerned about your weight, you should compare products based on both calories and fat. If you have heart disease or high blood pressure, you should focus on the amount of total fat, saturated fat, trans fat, cholesterol, and sodium. Choose products containing less than 20 percent daily values for fat, cholesterol, and sodium.

If you have diabetes, you should pay attention to the amount of sugar added to foods, as well as fiber. And follow these tips from the American Diabetes Association:

◆ Sugar-free does not mean carbohydrate-free. Compare the total carbohydrate content of a sugar-free food with that of the standard product. If there is a big difference in carbohydrate content between the two foods, you may want to buy the sugar-free food. If there is little difference in the total grams of carbohydrate between the two foods, choose the one you want based on price and taste. Make sure to read the label carefully to make the best choice.

◆ "No sugar added" foods do not have any form of sugar added during processing or packaging, and do not contain high-sugar ingredients. But they may still be high in carbohydrate, so you have to check the label.

◆ Fat-free foods can be higher in carbohydrate and contain almost the same calories as the foods they replace. One good example of this is fat-free cookies. Fat-free foods are not necessarily a better choice than the standard product, so read your labels carefully.

What Are Genetically Modified (GM) Foods?

Some products have GMO listed on them with a slash through the middle. They are controversial. But what are they? Genetic modification is a special set of technologies that change the genetic makeup of such living organisms as animals, plants, or bacteria.

Combining genes from different organisms is known as "recombinant DNA technology," and the resulting organism is said to be "genetically modified," "genetically engineered," or "transgenic." GM products (current or in the pipeline) include medicines and vaccines, foods and food ingredients, feeds, and fibers.

Locating genes for important traits—such as those conferring insect resistance or desired nutrients—is one of the most limiting steps in the process.

In 2003, about 167 million acres (67.7 million hectares) grown by 7 million farmers in 18 countries were planted with transgenic crops, the principal ones being herbicide- and insecticide-resistant soybeans, corn, cotton, and canola. Other crops include sweet potatoes, and rice with increased iron and other vitamins. Coming soon are bananas that produce human vaccines against infectious diseases such as hepatitis B; fish that mature more quickly; and fruit and nut trees that bear fruit much earlier than the "natural."

There are a number of major concerns about GM products, but two stand out. One concern is that genetically modifying crops could produce toxins. Another is that the introduction of any gene might cause an allergic reaction in some people. Advocates for GM say the process

For Crops:

◆ Enhances taste and quality.

◆ Reduces the time it takes for the crop to mature.

◆ Increases nutrients, yields, and stress tolerance.

◆ Improves resistance to disease, pests, and herbicides.

For Animals:

◆ Increases resistance, productivity, hardiness, and feed efficiency.

◆ Produces better yields of meat, eggs, and milk.

◆ Improves animal health and diagnostic methods.

For the Environment:

◆ Could produce herbicides and insecticides that are friendly to the environment.

◆ Conserves soil, water, and energy.

◆ Improves natural waste management.

◆ Results in more efficient processing.

For Society:

◆ Increases food security for growing populations.

Unfortunately, if you do not want to eat GMs you will not find any information about them on food labels. However, it is easier to find products that do not have them. They will say so.

Certifications Can Guide You to Health-Promoting Products

Looking for labels that certify that a food meets special qualifications can help assure you that you are getting what you think you are. (For information about the

Whole Grain Stamp, see Chapter 8.) Another important certification program is the American Heart Association's Heart-Check Mark. (In Canada, look for the Health Check.)

The American Heart Association established its Food Certification Program in 1995 to provide consumers an easy, reliable way to identify heart-healthy foods. To qualify, a food meets all of the following qualifying levels:

	Saturated Fat and Cholesterol	Saturated Fat, Cholesterol, and Whole Grains
Total fat	3 g or less	Less than 6.5 gms
Saturated fat	1 g or less	1 g or less
Cholesterol	20 mg or less	20 mg or less
Sodium	480 mg or less	480 mg or less
Contain 10% or more of the daily value of 1 of 6 nutrients: vitamin A, vitamin C, iron, calcium, protein, or dietary fiber	Yes	Yes
Trans fat.		.5 g or less
Whole grain		51% by weight/Reference Amount Customarily Consumed (RACC)
Minimum Dietary Fiber		1.7 g/RACC of 30 gms 2.5 g/RACC of 45 gs 2.8 g/RACC of 50 gs 3.0 g/RACC of 55 gs

Seafood, game meat, meat and poultry must meet the standards for "extra lean."

Reducing Food Contamination from Packaging

Chemicals in paper and plastics can transfer into food. It is important to eliminate the circumstances that can cause such migrations. The following tips can help you avoid corruption of your groceries from packaging.

◆ Plastic tends to contaminate fatty foods, especially hot fatty foods. Cool leftovers before placing in plastic storage containers.

◆ Plastic wrap should not come into direct contact with fatty foods in your microwave. Do not use plastic containers such as old yogurt tubs in the microwave. Always use ceramic or glass cookware instead.

◆ Be cautious of foods sold in microwavable packages. The chemical polyethylene terephthalate (PET) and adhesives can migrate from the packaging into the food.

◆ Be cautious about using plasticware when eating fatty foods.

◆ Do not use bleached paper products for coffee filters or other foods or drinks.

Conversion Guides

You may want to copy this table and always have it with your shopping list, so that you can make quick conversions when reading labels.

U.S. to Metric

Capacity

$^1/_5$ tsp. = 1 ml

1 tsp. = 5 ml

1 TB. = 15 ml

1 fluid oz. = 30 ml

$^1/_5$ cup = 50 ml

1 cup = 240 ml

2 cups (1 pint) = 470 ml

4 cups (1 quart) = .95 liter

4 quarts (1 gal.) = 3.8 liters

Weight

1 oz. = 28 grams

1 lb. = 454 grams

Metric to U.S.

Capacity

1 ml = $^1/_5$ tsp.
5 ml = 1 tsp.
15 ml = 1 TB.
30 ml = 1 fluid oz.
100 ml = 3.4 fluid oz.
240 ml = 1 cup
1 l = 34 fluid oz.
1 l = 4.2 cups
1 l = 2.1 pints
1 l = 1.06 quarts
1 l = .26 gallon

Weight

1 g = .035 oz.
100 g = 3.5 oz.
500 g = 1.10 lb.
1 kg = 2.205 lb.
1 kg = 35 oz.

Cooking Measurement Equivalents

16 TB. = 1 cup
12 TB. = ¾ cup
10 TB. + 2 tsp. = $^2/_3$ cup
8 TB. = ½ cup
6 TB. = $^3/_8$ cup
5 TB. + 1 tsp. = $^1/_3$ cup
4 TB. = ¼ cup
2 TB. = $^1/_8$ cup
2 TB. + 2 teaspoons = $^1/_6$ cup
1 TB. = $^1/_{16}$ cup

Cooking Measurement Equivalents
2 cups = 1 pint
2 pints = 1 quart
3 tsp. = 1 TB.
48 tsp. = 1 cup

The Least You Need to Know

◆ Fill your grocery cart about two thirds with fruits and vegetables.

◆ Make a list organized around health-promoting categories.

◆ Read nutrition labels to stay on track.

◆ Look for certification stamps, such as Heart-Check and others.

Chapter 15

Herbs and Supplements

In This Chapter

◆ Learn about supplements and the Food and Drug Administration

◆ Read what studies show about some popular supplements

◆ Understand the importance of taking a daily vitamin

In addition to following the seven principles of the anti-inflammation diet, you may be considering supplements such as multivitamins, herbs, or over-the-counter drugs to help with an inflammatory condition. (For information about the medications used to treat inflammation, see Chapter 1.) With some exceptions, this is a controversial area.

Because many products are marketed as dietary supplements, it is important to know what is in them and what their effects might be. Some supplements are extremely valuable because they help ensure that you get adequate amounts of essential nutrients or help promote optimal health and performance. Others are downright dangerous.

Supplements: What Is the Word?

Dietary supplements are big business, and there are many different types on the market. Now that inflammation is such a hot topic you will see more and more supplements advertised that claim to make you feel better. Often there is little, if any, scientific support for these claims.

Supplements may have vitamins, minerals, fiber, amino acids, herbs, or even hormones in them. They may be pills, capsules, powders, gel tabs, extracts, or liquids. And you don't even need a prescription from your doctor to buy dietary supplements.

However, in some cases, supplements have unwanted effects. Always check with your doctor or other qualified health-care provider before taking a supplement, especially when combining or substituting them with other foods or medicine.

So Much for Science

Some vitamins, minerals, and herbs have been scientifically studied; many have not. This is in large part because the U.S. Food and Drug Administration (FDA) does not have the authority to study and regulate them. Research studies on supplements to prove that they are effective and safe are not required before they are marketed. It is up to the manufacturers and distributors to make sure that their products are safe and that their label claims are accurate and truthful.

The FDA takes action against the manufacturer and/or distributor only if a supplement has been found to be dangerous after it is on the market. Supplements are being heavily studied by the FDA, other government agencies, and the National Academy of Sciences (NAS), while many private groups are interested in and studying dietary supplements as well.

Because of the lack of scrutiny, supplements can be a waste of money because they don't really help your problem. For example, taking antioxidants in supplement form has not been found in clinical trials to be effective.

 InflamWarnings _____

Sometimes a particular supplement does not have the ingredients that they claim. For example, scientists at the Good Housekeeping Institute analyzed eight brands of SAM-e, an herbal preparation sometimes touted as a "natural Prozac" to relieve depression, and found that two had only half the promised levels of active ingredient, and, incredibly, another had none at all. Consumer Reports also examined 10 brands of ginseng and concluded that several contained almost none of the active ingredient.

What is a consumer to do? Fortunately, the National Center for Complementary and Alternative Medicine (NCCAM) and other agencies have studied some of the most botanical popular supplements used for inflammatory conditions. The following sections cover what we know about them.

Thunder God Vine

Thunder god vine (TGV) is a perennial vine native to China, Japan, and Korea. Preparations made from the skinned root of TGV have been used in traditional Chinese medicine to treat inflammatory and autoimmune diseases. Interestingly, TGV also has been used to kill insects in farm fields.

TGV was studied by the University of Texas Southwestern Medical Center and the National Institutes of Health (NIH). People who participated had rheumatoid arthritis (RA). Twenty-one patients for whom conventional treatment had not worked completed the trial. Eighty percent of those who received a high-dose TGV extract and 40 percent of those who received a low-dose TGV extract experienced improvement in RA symptoms and physical functioning, while no one in the placebo group improved. However, the NCCAM urges that longer and larger studies are needed to confirm these findings and to find out more about TGV.

Parts of the TGV plant are dangerous. The leaves, the flowers, the main stem, and the skin covering the root are poisonous, to a point that they could cause death. You should never try to make TGV medications yourself.

Currently, there are no consistent, high-quality TGV products being manufactured in the United States. Preparations of TGV made outside the United States (for example, in China) can sometimes be obtained, but it is not possible to verify whether they are safe and effective.

If taken for a long time, TGV may deplete minerals in women's bones, which is especially important if you have osteoporosis or are at risk for it. If taken at high doses, TGV could suppress the immune system and increase the effects of immune-suppressing drugs.

GLA: Evening Primrose, Borage, and Black Currant

GLA (gamma-linolenic acid) is an omega-6 fatty acid found in the oils of some plant seeds, including evening primrose, borage, and black currant. Your body can use GLA to make anti-inflammatory substances. A review of seven studies on GLA (from evening primrose, borage, and black currant oils) suggests that it could provide relief for pain, morning stiffness, and joint tenderness in people with rheumatoid arthritis.

However, there are potential side effects and risks to know about with GLA. These plant seed oils may affect certain medical conditions and interact with prescription medications. Specifically, National Center for Complementary and Alternative Medicine (NCCAM) warns:

◆ Some borage seed oil preparations contain ingredients called PAs (for pyrrolizidine alkaloids) that can harm the liver or worsen liver disease. Only preparations that are certified and labeled as "PA-free" should be used.

◆ Borage oil and evening primrose oil might increase the risk of bleeding and bruising, especially in people taking blood-thinning drugs, such as aspirin, clopidogrel, NSAIDs, or warfarin.

◆ Evening primrose oil may cause problems for people taking a class of psychiatric drugs called phenothiazines, such as chlorpromazine or prochlorperazine.

Side effects of these oils can include nausea, diarrhea, soft stool, intestinal gas, burping, and stomach bloating.

Fish Oil

Fish oil contains high amounts of two omega-3 fatty acids: EPA (eicosapentaenoic acid) and DHA (docosahexaenoic acid) (see Chapter 7). As with GLA, the body can use omega-3s to make substances that reduce inflammation.

There is some encouraging evidence from a number of laboratory studies, animal studies, and clinical trials about the potential usefulness of fish-oil supplements. However, more research is needed to definitively answer various questions, including what the most effective dosage or length of treatment is.

 InflamWarnings _____

In some people, the high amounts of omega-3s that are present in fish oil can increase the risk of bleeding or affect the time it takes blood to clot. If a person is taking drugs that affect bleeding or is going to have surgery, this is of special concern. Fish-oil supplements interact with medicines for high blood pressure, so taking them together might lower a person's blood pressure too much.

There are several points to remember about fish-oil capsules:

◆ Certain species of fish can contain high levels of contaminants, such as mercury, from the environment (see Chapter 7).

◆ Another point to note about safety is that a product called fish liver oil can contain more vitamin A than the recommended daily dosage, which could cause problems.

◆ Side effects may include a fishy aftertaste, belching, stomach disturbances, and nausea.

Valerian

The herb valerian is used for problems with sleep and anxiety disorders, which can occur for some people who have inflammatory problems. Valerian is also taken to relieve muscle and joint pain. The species of valerian most used in American supplements is *Valeriana officinalis*.

Analysis by the NCCAM suggests that valerian has at least mild benefits for insomnia. There is not much evidence on how long it is safe to take valerian and what dose to use.

There is also not enough reliable evidence to know whether valerian is effective for muscle and joint pain, including pain from RA. There is some evidence that it could be helpful for musculoskeletal pain.

Valerian is considered generally safe with some exceptions.

 InflamWarnings

Valerian should not be taken with sedatives (for example, alcohol, benzodiazepines, or narcotics) or sedative herbs (such as melatonin, SAM-e, or St. John's wort). Valerian increases sedative effects.

People who are taking antifungal drugs, statins, or certain antiarrhythmia drugs also should not take valerian. Valerian may not be safe for people who have a liver disorder or are at risk for one. After taking valerian, caution should be used in driving or using dangerous machinery. Side effects of valerian can include drowsiness in the morning, headache, stomach problems, excitability or anxiety, and sleeplessness.

Other Botanicals

Three other botanicals claim to benefit inflammatory arthritis:

◆ Ginger

◆ Curcumin (a component of the spice turmeric)

◆ Boswellia (also called Indian frankincense, made from the resin of a tree that grows in India)

These three botanicals have a history of use in the ancient Hindu science of health and medicine, Ayurveda, to treat inflammatory conditions. Because some earlier studies showed promise, NCCAM is sponsoring studies at the University of Arizona on these three botanicals.

A fourth botanical, feverfew, has been used in folk medicine with an intent to treat arthritis, migraine, and other conditions. The NCCAM identified only one study of feverfew and found no more benefit from feverfew than from the placebo.

Ginger's possible side effects include stomach upset, diarrhea, and irritation to the mouth and throat.

Curcumin can have side effects of stomach problems, including nausea and diarrhea. Curcumin could add to the effects of other herbs and drugs that slow blood clotting. Curcumin can also cause gallbladder contractions and should not be used by people with gallbladder disease or gallstones.

Boswellia can have side effects of stomach pain, stomach upset, nausea, and diarrhea. It is not known whether boswellia interacts with any drugs, supplements, or diseases and conditions.

Feverfew appears to be safe for short-term use, but the safety of long-term use is not known. Feverfew can cause an allergic reaction, especially in people who are allergic to the daisy family. Side effects can include diarrhea and other stomach upsets. Chewing fresh leaves of feverfew may cause mouth irritation and sores. Feverfew might interact with medications broken down by the liver and increase the actions of drugs that slow blood clotting. Pregnant women should not take feverfew.

InflamWarnings

Ginger is not recommended for people who have a bleeding disorder, a heart condition, or diabetes. Ginger may further slow blood clotting when combined with other herbs and drugs that slow blood clotting; add to the blood-pressure-lowering effects of drugs for high blood pressure and heart disease; and add to the blood-sugar-lowering effects of diabetes drugs.

Glucosamine and Chondroitin

Glucosamine sulfate (glucosamine for short) and chondroitin sulfate (chondroitin) are popular dietary supplements for arthritis. You can buy them separately, in combination with each other, and in other combinations.

Glucosamine is a substance found in the fluid around the joints. It can also be obtained from the shells of shrimp, lobster, and crabs, or made in the laboratory. Our bodies make glucosamine to make and repair cartilage, a firm but flexible tissue that covers the ends of bones, keeps them from rubbing against each other, and absorbs the force of impact.

Chondroitin is a substance found in the cartilage around joints. As a supplement, it is obtained from sources such as sharks and cattle.

Glucosamine/chondroitin was the subject of a large clinical trial in the United States called GAIT. The University of Utah School of Medicine coordinated this study, which was conducted at 16 rheumatology research centers across the United States. The primary outcome of the study was that users of glucosamine/chondroitin had at least a 20 percent reduction in pain at 24 weeks.

Glucosamine appears to be safe for most people with some exceptions.

 InflamWarnings

Glucosamine can worsen asthma through an allergic reaction. Also, glucosamine might cause higher blood sugar and insulin levels in people with diabetes, and those who decide to use it need to carefully monitor their blood sugar. Glucosamine could possibly decrease the effectiveness of certain medications—acetaminophen, some anticancer drugs, and antidiabetes drugs.

Generally, side effects of glucosamine can include mild stomach problems and nausea; less commonly, there can be sleepiness, a skin reaction, or a headache. Some people who are allergic to shellfish are concerned about an allergic reaction to glucosamine. However, most shellfish allergies are to proteins in the meat, not to the shell material from which glucosamine supplements are made.

Chondroitin appears to be safe for most people. However, chondroitin may possibly worsen asthma (through an allergic response), blood clotting disorders, and prostate cancer.

The side effects of chondroitin can include stomach pain and nausea, and, less commonly, diarrhea, constipation, swelling, and problems with heart rate.

Both supplements could affect the action of the drug warfarin, but this is not definite.

SAM-e

SAM-e is an amino acid product that some people take because they believe that it improves brain and joint function. The federal Agency for Healthcare Research and Quality (AHRQ) conducted an analysis of published literature to evaluate whether the supplement SAM-e is effective and safe. A panel of technical experts representing diverse disciplines was established to advise the researchers throughout the research. SAM-e was found to be effective in helping with the pain of arthritis and even had a positive impact on depression. However, SAM-e was not any more effective than taking an NSAID (see Chapter 1).

Ginkgo

Ginkgo seeds have been used in traditional Chinese medicine for thousands of years. More recently, ginkgo leaf extract has been used to treat asthma, bronchitis, fatigue, and tinnitus (ringing in the ears).

Today, people use ginkgo leaf extracts hoping to improve memory; to treat or help prevent Alzheimer's disease and other types of dementia; to decrease intermittent claudication (leg pain caused by narrowing arteries); and to treat sexual dysfunction, multiple sclerosis, tinnitus, and other health conditions. Ginkgo can be found in tablets, capsules, or teas. Occasionally, ginkgo extracts are used in skin products.

Numerous studies of ginkgo have been done with mixed results. Some promising results have been seen for Alzheimer's disease/dementia, intermittent claudication, and tinnitus among others, but larger, well-designed research studies are needed. NCCAM is presently conducting a large clinical trial of ginkgo with more than 3,000 volunteers.

Side effects of ginkgo may include headache, nausea, gastrointestinal upset, diarrhea, dizziness, or allergic skin reactions. More severe allergic reactions have occasionally been reported.

Quercetin

Quercetin, which is primarily found in apples, onions, and black tea, is a type of flavonoid (plant pigment) that serves as a building block for other members of the flavonoid family. It is thought to have strong anti-inflammatory properties. However, quercetin as a supplement has not been rigorously studied and it's too early to recommend it as a supplement. It is better to get it from apples and other foods.

> **InflamWarnings**
>
> The results of some studies suggest that ginkgo can increase the risk of bleeding, so if you take anticoagulant drugs, have bleeding disorders, or have scheduled surgery or dental procedures, you should use caution and talk to a health care provider if you are using ginkgo.
>
> Uncooked ginkgo seeds contain a chemical known as ginkgotoxin, which can cause seizures. Consuming large quantities of seeds over time can cause death. Ginkgo leaf and ginkgo leaf extracts appear to contain little ginkgotoxin.

Don't take quercetin if you take the calcium channel blocker felodipine for high blood pressure. In test-tube studies, quercetin inhibited enzymes that break down felodipine; in theory this could increase blood levels of the drug and lead to unwanted side effects.

Antioxidants

There is no proof that large doses of antioxidants will prevent inflammatory diseases such as heart disease or diabetes. Eating a lot of fruits and vegetables rather than taking a supplement is the best way to get antioxidants. Vegetable oil and nuts are also good sources of some antioxidants. Nondairy calcium sources are especially good for people who cannot use dairy products.

Tips from the National Institutes of Health

If you are thinking about using supplements for any reason, remember:

◆ Talk to your doctor or a registered dietitian. Just because something worked for your neighbor doesn't mean the same will be true for you.

◆ Use only the supplement your doctor or dietitian and you decide on—don't buy combinations that have things you don't want or need.

◆ If your doctor does not suggest a dietary supplement, but you decide to use one anyway, still let your doctors and other health providers know. Then they can keep an eye on your health and adjust your other medications if needed.

♦ Learn as much as you can about the supplement you are thinking about, but be aware of the source of the information. Could the writer or group profit from the sale of a particular supplement?

InflamWarnings

Remember, if you see a product advertised as "natural," it does not necessarily mean that it is "safe" or that it even does what it suggests that it will do.

♦ Buy brands you know from companies you, your doctor, dietitian, or pharmacist know are reputable.

♦ Remember that many of the claims made about supplements are not based on enough scientific proof. If you have questions about a supplement, contact the firm and ask if it has information on the safety and/or effectiveness of the ingredients in its product.

Hormones, Aging, and Inflammation

Hormones are one of the most common and vital chemical messengers in the body. Although some proponents are convinced that hormone supplements can reverse aging and inflammation, there is little scientific evidence for this claim.

For more than a decade, the National Institute on Aging (NIA) has supported and conducted studies of replenishing hormones to find out if they may help reduce frailty and improve function in older people. These studies have focused on hormones known to decline as we grow older, including:

♦ Dehydroepiandrosterone (DHEA)

♦ Growth hormone

♦ Melatonin

Some of these hormones are available over the counter and can be used without consulting a physician. The federal National Institutes of Health (NIA), which studies these hormones, does not recommend taking them as an "anti-aging" remedy because they have not been proven to serve this purpose. And the influence of these supplements on a person's health is unknown, particularly when taken over a long period of time.

The following information on these hormones is from NIA.

DHEA

Dehydroepiandrosterone is made from cholesterol by the adrenal glands, which sit on top of each kidney.

Production of this substance peaks in the mid-20s, and gradually declines with age in most people. What this drop means or how it affects the aging process, if at all, is unclear. However, researchers do know that the body converts DHEA into two hormones that are known to affect us in many ways: estrogen and testosterone (see below).

Supplements of DHEA can be bought without a prescription and are sold as "anti-aging remedies." Some proponents of these products claim that DHEA supplements improve energy, strength, and immunity. DHEA is also said to increase muscle and decrease fat.

At present there is no consistent evidence that DHEA supplements do any of these things in people, and there is little scientific evidence to support the use of DHEA as a "rejuvenating" hormone. Although the long-term (over 1 year) effects of DHEA supplements have not been studied, there are early signs that they can cause physical harm, including liver damage.

In addition, NIA points out that some people's bodies make more estrogen and testosterone from DHEA than others. There is no way to predict who will make more and who will make less.

Researchers are concerned that DHEA supplements may cause high levels of estrogen or testosterone in some people. This is important because testosterone may play a role in prostate cancer, and higher levels of estrogen are associated with an increased risk of breast cancer. It is not yet known for certain if supplements of estrogen and testosterone, or supplements of DHEA, also increase the risk of developing these types of cancer. In women, high testosterone levels can cause acne and growth of facial hair.

Overall, the studies that have been done so far do not provide a clear picture of the risks and benefits of DHEA. For example, some studies in older people show that DHEA helps build muscle and reduce fat, but other studies do not.

Growth Hormone

Human growth hormone (hGH) is made by the pituitary gland, a pea-sized structure located at the base of the brain, and is important for normal development and maintenance of tissues and organs. It is especially important for normal growth in children.

Studies have shown that injections of supplemental hGH are helpful to certain people. Sometimes children are unusually short because their bodies do not make enough hGH. When they receive injections of this hormone, their growth improves. Young adults who have no pituitary gland (because of surgery for a pituitary tumor, for example) cannot make the hormone and they become obese. When they are given hGH, they lose weight.

Like some other hormones, blood levels of hGH often decrease as people age, but this may not necessarily be bad. At least one epidemiological study, for instance, suggests that people who have high levels of hGH are more apt to die at younger ages than those with lower levels of the hormone. Studies of animals with genetic disorders that suppress growth hormone production and secretion also suggest that *reduced* growth hormone secretion may prolong survival in some species.

Although there is no conclusive evidence that hGH can prevent aging, some people spend a great deal of money on supplements. These supplements are claimed by some to increase muscle, decrease fat, and to boost an individual's stamina and sense of well-being. Shots—the only proven way of getting the body to make use of supplemental hGH—can cost more than $15,000 a year. They are available only by prescription and should be given by a doctor. Some dietary supplements, known as human growth hormone releasers, are marketed as a low-cost alternative to hGH shots. But claims that these over-the-counter products retard the aging process are unsubstantiated.

Although some studies have shown that supplemental hGH does increase muscle mass, it seems to have little impact on muscle strength or function. Scientists are continuing to study hGH, but they are watching their study participants very carefully because side effects can be serious in older adults. These include diabetes and pooling of fluid in the skin and other tissues, which may lead to high blood pressure and heart failure. Joint pain and carpal tunnel syndrome also may occur.

A recent report that treatment of children with human pituitary growth hormone increases the risk of subsequent cancer is a cause for concern. Further studies on this issue are needed. Whether older people treated with hGH for extended periods have an increased risk of cancer is unknown.

For now, there is no convincing evidence hGH supplements will improve the health of those who do not suffer a profound deficiency of this hormone.

Melatonin

Melatonin is a hormone that is made by the pineal gland, a structure in the brain. Contrary to the claims of some, secretion of melatonin does not necessarily decrease with age. Instead, a number of factors, including light and many common medications, can affect melatonin secretion in people of any age.

Melatonin supplements can be bought without a prescription.

Claims that melatonin can slow or reverse aging are very far from proven. Studies of melatonin have been much too limited to support these claims and have focused on animals, not people.

Research on sleep shows that melatonin does play a role in our daily sleep/wake cycle, and that supplements, in amounts ranging from 0.1 to 0.5 milligrams, can improve sleep in some cases.

If melatonin is taken at the wrong time, though, it can disrupt the sleep/wake cycle. Other side effects may include confusion, drowsiness, and headache the next morning.

What About Vitamins and Minerals?

The best way to get vitamins and minerals is through the foods you eat. However, taking a daily multivitamin can be great insurance when you are not always able to eat as many nutrients as you need to.

Dr. Walter Willett from the Harvard Medical School, whom we have mentioned throughout this book, and his staff recommend taking a standard multivitamin daily, although he emphasizes that a supplement doesn't come close to making up for an unhealthy diet. Willett says, "It provides a dozen or so of the vitamins known to maintain health, a mere shadow of what's available from eating plenty of fruits, vegetables, and whole grains. Instead, a daily multivitamin provides a sort of nutritional safety net."

Dr. Willet says that a standard RDA-level (recommended dietary allowance) multivitamin can supply you with enough of these vitamins for under $40 a year.

The NAS has developed recommendations for vitamins and minerals (check the list in Chapter 14). Be sure to check the label on your supplement bottle. It shows the level of vitamins and minerals in a serving compared with the suggested daily intake for a person eating 2,000 calories a day. For example, a vitamin A intake of 100 percent DV (daily value) means the supplement is giving you the full amount of vitamin A you need each day. This is in addition to what you are getting from your food.

Keep Track of Everything You Take

Supplements can act like drugs in your body and interact with other medicines that you take, all of which can greatly affect your health. It is important that your health provider be aware of everything you take, *including supplements*. Follow these tips adapted from the National Institutes of Health:

- Make a list of all the medicines and supplements you take. Show it to all your health-care providers, including physical therapists and dentists. Keep one copy in your medicine cabinet and one in your wallet or pocketbook. The list should include the name of each medicine, doctor who prescribed it, reason it was prescribed, amount you take, and time(s) you take it.

InflamWarnings

Depending on the supplement—and your age, weight, and health— taking more than 100 percent DV of a vitamin or mineral could be harmful to your health. And large doses of some vitamins and minerals can also keep your pre- scription medications from work- ing as they should.

- Read and save all written information that comes with the medicine.

- Take your medicine in the exact amount and at the time your doctor prescribes.

- Call your doctor right away if you have any problems with your medicine or if you are wor- ried that the medicine might be doing more harm than good. Your doctor may be able to change your medicine to a different one that will work better for you.

- Use a memory aid to take your medicines on time. Some people use meals or bedtime as reminders to take their medicine. Other people use charts, calendars, and weekly pill boxes to remind them. Use a system that works for you.

  Do not skip doses of medication or take half doses to save money. Talk with your doctor or pharmacist if you can't afford the prescribed medicine. There may be less costly choices or special programs to help with the cost of certain drugs.

- Avoid mixing alcohol and medicine. Some medicines may not work correctly or may make you sick if taken with alcohol.

- Take your medicine until it's finished or until your doctor says it's okay to stop.

- Don't take medicines prescribed for another person or give yours to someone else.

- Don't take medicine in the dark. To avoid making a mistake, turn your light on before reaching for your pills.

- Check the expiration dates on your medicine bottles and throw away outdated medicines.

◆ Don't leave your medicine on a kitchen table or counter where a young child may get into it. Make sure you store all medicines and supplements out of sight and out of reach of children.

◆ Remember, medicines that are strong enough to cure you can also be strong enough to hurt you if they aren't used the right way.

The Least You Need to Know

◆ Make sure you know what is in any supplement you take.

◆ Remember many supplements have not been studied for effectiveness and safety. The same is true for herbs.

◆ Make a list of all the medications and supplements you take.

◆ Share your list with your health providers.

◆ Take a multivitamin every day.

Part 4

Exercise and Stress Reduction

Inflammation can cause stress and other physical problems. In turn, many people respond to the pain and stress that accompany inflammation by not getting adequate exercise. And, ironically, not exercising is one of the worst things you can do for your body. Among other things, it can lead to metabolic syndrome, a major cause of inflammation.

In these chapters, we show you how to reduce stress (including how to quit smoking if that is a problem for you) and get exercise to move forward in your life and cut down on the negative effects of inflammation.

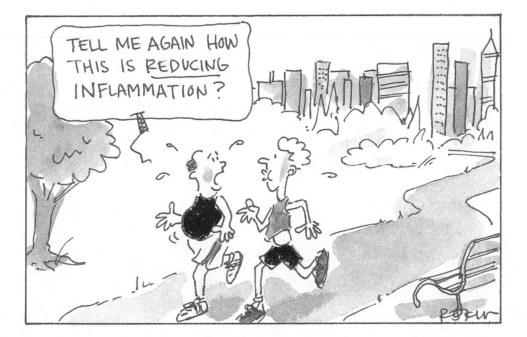

16

Stress Reduction

In This Chapter

◆ Understand the signs of stress

◆ Learn tips on how to relax

◆ Learn tips on how to quit smoking

We all have stress in our lives. Stress is the result of how we react to events in our world. It's the fight-or-flight instinct that is the body's way of facing down challenges. These challenges can be real or in our minds—our bodies react the same way.

Inflammation can cause pain and other physical problems, which create challenges in their own right. Your body responds to these stressors by calling your nervous system and specific hormones into action.

This chapter provides techniques, such as meditation and progressive relaxation, to help you reduce stress. And because smoking is an all-too-frequent and dangerous response to stress, we offer some tips on how to quit for those who need them.

What Is Stress?

When stress occurs in response to a challenge, your body releases hormones into your bloodstream. These hormones speed up your heart and breathing and other physical processes. Even your liver gets into the act. It releases some of its stored glucose to give your body energy to fight the challenge. Among other things, your muscles tighten. You produce sweat to cool your body. All of these physical changes prepare you to react fast. This natural reaction is known as the *stress response*.

Stress doesn't occur just in response to immediate challenges. Long-term challenges, like coping with an illness, can produce a low-level, long-term stress that wears people down.

def•i•ni•tion

A **stress response** is the physical and mental change that occurs due to stress. For example, sweating, an increased heart beat, and feelings of anxiety can be stress responses.

Signs of Stress

If you are experiencing stress, you may have one of the following signs:

- Anxiety or panic attacks
- Feeling pressured, hassled, and hurried
- Irritability and moodiness
- Physical symptoms, such as stomach problems, headaches, or even chest pain
- Allergic reactions, such as eczema or asthma
- Problems sleeping
- Drinking too much, smoking, overeating, or doing drugs
- Sadness or depression

The Different Kinds of Stress

According to the American Psychological Association, there are different types of stress—acute stress, episodic acute stress, and chronic stress—each with its own characteristics, symptoms, duration, and treatment approaches.

Acute stress is the most common form. It comes from demands and pressures of the recent past and anticipated demands and pressures of the near future. Fortunately, because it is short term, acute stress doesn't have enough time to do the extensive damage associated with long-term stress.

Episodic acute stress occurs when acute stresses occur often. This usually occurs for "Type A" personalities, first described by cardiologists Meyer Friedman and Ray Rosenman. Type As have an "excessive competitive drive, aggressiveness, impatience, and a harrying sense of time urgency."

Chronic stress is the grinding stress that wears people away day after day, year after year. Chronic stress may damage bodies, minds, and lives, and it comes when a person never sees a way out of a miserable situation.

Another form of chronic stress comes from ceaseless worry. Worrywarts see disaster around every corner and pessimistically forecast catastrophe in every situation.

Coping with Stress

There are a number of methods for learning how to manage the stress that comes along with any new challenge, good or bad. Some of the things at the top of the list are:

- ◆ Learn to relax. The body's natural antidote to stress is called the relaxation response. It is the opposite of stress, and it creates a sense of well-being and calm.

- ◆ Get enough sleep to keep your body and mind in top shape, making you more able to cope with pain and challenges.

- ◆ Check your attitude. Your outlook, attitude, and thoughts influence the way you see things.

- ◆ Get regular exercise (see Chapter 17).

- ◆ Eat nourishing food (follow the seven principles of the anti-inflammation diet).

- ◆ Maintain a healthy weight.

- ◆ Don't smoke!

Meditation

Meditation is a group of techniques, most of which started in Eastern religious or spiritual traditions. Today, many people use meditation outside of its traditional religious or cultural settings, for health and wellness purposes. When meditating you focus your attention and quiet the thoughts that normally occupy your mind.

No one knows for sure how it works, but for many people it leads to a state of greater physical relaxation, mental calmness, and psychological balance. Practicing meditation can change how you relate to the flow of emotions and thoughts in the mind.

Meditation usually has four elements in common:

◆ A quiet location. Many meditators prefer a quiet place with as few distractions as possible.

◆ A specific, comfortable posture. Depending on the type being practiced, meditation can be done while sitting, lying down, standing, walking, or in other positions.

◆ A focus of attention. Focusing one's attention is usually a part of meditation. For example, the meditator may focus on a mantra (a specially chosen word or set of words), an object, or the act of breathing.

◆ An open attitude. Having an open attitude during meditation means letting distractions come and go naturally without stopping to think about them. When distracting or wandering thoughts occur, they are not suppressed; instead, the meditator gently brings attention back to the focus.

Meditation is practiced both on its own and as a component of some other therapies, such as yoga, tai chi, and qi gong. Practicing meditation has been shown to induce some changes in the body, such as changes in the body's "fight or flight" response.

InflamWise

The Chinese practice of tai chi has become a popular way to reduce stress and build agility. This meditation-in-motion technique is a gentle exercise in which you perform no strenuous action. The slow, synchronized movements of tai chi are easy to learn and perform.

Instruction of tai chi is now available in most communities. The program is so effective that it has been endorsed by the Arthritis Foundation as a way to cope with pain. Instruction videos are also available.

Using Meditation to Relax

With the following meditation technique, you repeat words or suggestions in your mind to help you relax and reduce the tension in your muscles. This technique is also a great way of reducing negative thoughts and creating a positive attitude. Here is the basic technique:

1. Find a peaceful place where you'll be free of interruptions. Choose a focus word, phrase, or image you find relaxing. Examples of words or phrases include "grace" or "I am relaxed."

2. Sit quietly in a comfortable position.

3. Close your eyes and relax your muscles, starting at your head, working down your body to your feet.

4. Breathe slowly and naturally, focusing on your word, phrase, or image. Continue for 10 to 20 minutes. If your mind wanders, that's okay. Gently return your focus to your breathing and the word, phrase, or image you selected.

5. After time is up, sit quietly for a few minutes with your eyes closed. Open your eyes and sit in silence for a few more minutes.

Relaxed Breathing

Stress causes rapid, shallow breathing. This kind of breathing sustains other aspects of the stress response, such as rapid heart rate and perspiration. If you can get control of your breath, the effects of acute stress become less intense.

There are a number of techniques for practicing relaxed breathing. Here is one tried-and-true approach:

1. Inhale. With your mouth closed and your shoulders relaxed, inhale as slowly and deeply as you can to the count of six. As you do that, push your stomach out. Allow the air to fill your diaphragm.

2. Hold. Keep the air in your lungs as you slowly count to four.

3. Exhale. Release the air through your mouth as you slowly count to six.

4. Repeat. Complete the inhale-hold-exhale cycle three to five times.

Progressive Muscle Relaxation

Progressive muscle relaxation can reduce the tightness in your muscles. Here is the basic technique:

◆ Find a quiet place where you won't be distracted.

◆ Make sure that your clothing is comfortable. Remove your glasses or contacts if you'd like.

◆ Tense each muscle group for at least 5 seconds and then relax for at least 30 seconds. Repeat before moving to the next muscle group.

And here is a basic walk-through of muscle relaxation:

1. Lift your eyebrows toward the ceiling, feeling the tension in your forehead and scalp. Relax. Repeat.

2. Squint your eyes tightly and wrinkle your nose and mouth, feeling the tension in the center of your face. Relax. Repeat.

3. Clench your teeth and pull back the corners of your mouth toward your ears. Show your teeth like a snarling dog. Relax. Repeat.

4. Gently touch your chin to your chest. Feel the pull in the back of your neck as it spreads into your head. Relax. Repeat.

5. Pull your shoulders up toward your ears, feeling the tension in your shoulders, head, neck, and upper back. Relax. Repeat.

6. Pull your arms back and press your elbows in toward the sides of your body. Try not to tense your lower arms. Feel the tension in your arms, shoulders, and into your back. Relax. Repeat.

7. Make a tight fist and pull up your wrists. Feel the tension in your hands, knuckles, and lower arms. Relax. Repeat.

8. Pull your shoulders back as if you're trying to make your shoulder blades touch. Relax. Repeat.

9. Pull your stomach in toward your spine, tightening your abdominal muscles. Relax. Repeat.

10. Squeeze your knees together and lift your legs up off the chair or from wherever you're relaxing. Feel the tension in your thighs. Relax. Repeat.

11. Raise your feet toward the ceiling while flexing them toward your body. Feel the tension in your calves. Relax. Repeat.

12. Turn your feet inward and curl your toes up and out. Relax. Repeat.

Listen to Soothing Sounds

Listening to soothing sounds can help ease daily tensions. There are three types of relaxation CDs or downloads that can help you relax. They include …

◆ Guided meditations.

◆ Narration to help with visualizing peaceful and safe imaginary places.

◆ Soothing music or nature sounds.

Yoga

Yoga is a specific system of exercises for reaching physical and mental control and well-being. It began more than 3,000 years ago in India. Yoga includes exercise and disciplining your mind and body to connect with your spirituality.

The physical part of yoga is called hatha yoga. Hatha yoga focuses on asanas, or poses. A person who practices yoga goes through a series of specific poses while controlling his or her breathing. Some types of yoga also involve meditation and chanting.

What the Experts Say

Today's yoga participants are young and old, flexible and inflexible, shapely and out of shape. They are everyday people just like you who want to treat their bodies well. And what better way than through a low-impact exercise that induces relaxation, lowers stress, and relieves tension? Even better, yoga also helps tone and strengthen your muscles and loosen your joints.

Source: Arthritis Foundation, *Let's Do Yoga*

There are many different types of hatha yoga:

◆ Ashtanga yoga is a vigorous, fast-paced yoga that helps to build flexibility, strength, concentration, and stamina. When doing Ashtanga yoga, you move quickly through a set of predetermined poses while remaining focused on deep breathing.

◆ Power yoga is similar to Ashtanga yoga and includes poses. This type of yoga is popular in the United States.

◆ Bikram yoga is also known as "hot yoga." It is practiced in rooms that may be heated to more than 100°F.

◆ Gentle yoga focuses on slow stretches, flexibility, and deep breathing.

◆ Kundalini yoga uses poses, deep breathing and other breathing techniques, chanting, and meditation.

◆ Iyengar yoga focuses on precise poses. Participants use benches, ropes, mats, blocks, and chairs.

Did You Know?

The stars do it.

Gwyneth Paltrow, David Duchovny, Julia Louis-Dreyfuss, Melissa Joan Hart, Jane Fonda, Angelina Jolie, Charlie Sheen, Sarah Jessica Parker, Kristin Davis, all three Dixie Chicks, and Kareem Abdul-Jabbar—what do these stars have in common?

They are all avid yoga practitioners.

Deep-Breathing Exercises

Deep breathing is another popular meditative technique that is very effective for relaxing. When you are stressed your breathing becomes shallow; this method helps you overcome that tendency. Here are some basic steps:

1. Lie down or sit in a comfortable chair, maintaining good posture. Your body should be as relaxed as possible. Close your eyes. Scan your body for tension.

2. Pay attention to how you are breathing. Place one hand on the part of your chest or abdomen that seems to rise and fall the most with each breath. If this spot is in your chest, you are not utilizing the lower part of your lungs.

3. Place both hands on your abdomen and follow your breathing, noticing how your abdomen rises and falls.

4. Breathe through your nose.

5. Notice if your chest is moving in harmony with your abdomen.

6. Now place one hand on your abdomen and one on your chest.

7. Inhale deeply and slowly through your nose into your abdomen. You should feel your abdomen rise with this inhalation and your chest should move only a little.

8. Exhale through your mouth, keeping your mouth, tongue, and jaw relaxed.

9. Relax as you focus on the sound and feeling of long, slow, deep breaths.

Quit It!

If you smoke, you have heard it all before. Smoking kills.

To remind you here are some facts about smoking from the Surgeon General's most recent report:

◆ Smoking harms nearly every organ of the body, causing many diseases and reducing the health of smokers in general.

◆ Quitting smoking has immediate as well as long-term benefits, reducing risks for diseases caused by smoking and improving health in general.

◆ Smoking cigarettes with low *tar* and *nicotine* provides no clear benefit to health.

def•i•ni•tion

Nicotine is a colorless, poisonous substance derived from the tobacco plant and used as an insecticide. It is the substance in tobacco to which smokers can become addicted.

Tar is the name for the substance produced by the burning of tobacco. Tar is purportedly the most destructive part of tobacco smoking, accumulating in the smoker's lungs over time and damaging them through various biochemical and mechanical processes.

The diseases caused by smoking include abdominal aortic aneurysm, acute myeloid leukemia, cataracts, cervical cancer, kidney cancer, pancreatic cancer, pneumonia, gum disease, stomach cancer, bladder cancer, esophageal cancer, laryngeal cancer, lung cancer, oral cancer, throat cancer, chronic lung diseases, and coronary heart and cardiovascular diseases, as well as reproductive problems.

InflamWarnings

Smoke from other people's cigarettes, known as secondhand smoke, causes cancer. There are more than 4,000 chemicals in secondhand smoke. More than 50
of these chemicals cause cancer in people or animals. Every year, about 3,000 non-
smokers die from lung cancer due to secondhand smoke.

Good News About Smoking

The good news about smoking is that many people have quit successfully. In fact,
every year more than 1 million smokers kick the habit. Many hospitals and community
centers offer programs in quitting smoking. Look in your local paper or yellow pages
or Google the phrase "quit smoking" and the name of your town.

Did You Know?

As a government looking out for the health of its citizens, New York City could become
a model for other areas of the country. Its Nicotine Replacement Therapy Giveaway
Program, sponsored by the New York City Department of Health and Mental Hygiene
(DOHMH), is giving away 35,000 courses of nicotine replacement therapy (NRT)
patches at no cost to smokers across the city who want to quit.

Eligible smokers receive four weeks of nicotine patches (21 mg), with the option to
receive an additional 2 weeks' worth (14 mg); instructions on how to use the patch;
and literature on how to quit smoking.

Five Keys for Quitting Smoking

Studies have shown that these five steps from the Centers for Disease Control (CDC)
will help you quit—and quit for good. You have the best chances of quitting if you use
them together:

- Get ready
- Get support
- Learn new skills and behaviors
- Get medication and use it correctly
- Be prepared for relapse or difficult situations

Details of these five steps are outlined in the next sections.

Get Ready

Here is step 1:

◆ Set a quit date.

◆ Change your environment.

◆ Get rid of all cigarettes and ashtrays in your home, car, and place of work.

◆ Don't let people smoke around you.

◆ Review your past attempts to quit. Think about what worked and what did not.

◆ After you quit, don't smoke—not even a puff!

Get Support and Encouragement

Studies have shown that you have a better chance of being successful if you have help. You can get support in many ways. Step 2 is:

◆ Tell your family, friends, and co-workers that you are going to quit and want their support. Ask them not to smoke around you or leave cigarettes out where you can see them.

◆ Talk to your health-care provider (doctor, dentist, nurse, pharmacist, psychologist, or smoking cessation coach or counselor).

◆ Get individual, group, or telephone counseling. Counseling doubles your chances of success.

◆ The more help you have, the better your chances are of quitting. Free programs are available at local hospitals and health centers. Call your local health department for information about programs in your area.

Learn New Skills and Behaviors

Step 3 is to try techniques that can replace your need to smoke. They include …

◆ Try to distract yourself from urges to smoke. Talk to someone, go for a walk, or get busy with a task.

◆ When you first try to quit, change your routine.

- Use a different route to work. Drink tea instead of coffee. Eat breakfast in a different place.

- Do something to reduce your stress. Take a hot bath, exercise, or read a book.

- Plan something enjoyable to do every day.

- Drink a lot of water and other fluids.

Get Medication and Use It Correctly

Medications can help you stop smoking and lessen the urge to smoke. The U.S. Food and Drug Administration (FDA) has approved six medications to help you quit smoking:

- Bupropion SR—available by prescription

- Nicotine gum—available over the counter

- Nicotine inhaler—available by prescription

- Nicotine nasal spray—available by prescription

- Nicotine patch—available by prescription and over the counter

- Nicotine lozenge—available over the counter

Ask your health-care provider for advice and carefully read the information on the package. All of these medications will double your chances of quitting, and quitting for good.

 InflamWise _____

One drug approved for smoking cessation differs from the others. It does not have nicotine as an ingredient. Bupropion SR (sustained-release) is a non-nicotine pill approved to treat tobacco dependence. It is also used as an antidepressant.

Bupropion treatment must be started before quitting smoking, as it helps prepare a smoker's body for the actual stress of quitting. Users are usually advised to begin taking bupropion approximately 1 to 2 weeks before they plan to quit. If you are planning on quitting smoking, you may want to ask your doctor or other health-care provider about it.

Nearly everyone who is trying to quit can benefit from using a medication. However, if you are pregnant or trying to become pregnant, nursing, under age 18, smoking fewer than 10 cigarettes per day, or have a medical condition, talk to your doctor or other health-care provider before taking medications.

InflamWise

Medicare will now cover smoking-cessation programs for some Medicare beneficiaries. The benefit is available for Medicare recipients who have an illness caused or complicated by tobacco use, including heart disease, cerebrovascular disease, lung disease, weak bones, blood clots, and cataracts. The bulk of Medicare spending today is for these diseases.

Smoking-cessation coverage is also available to beneficiaries who take any of many medications whose effectiveness is complicated by tobacco use, including insulins and medicines for high blood pressure, blood clots, and depression.

InflamWise

Check with your employer or health insurance plan to see if they offer smoking-cessation coverage. More and more employers are covering smoking-cessation. For example, the *Wall Street Journal* reports that Pennsylvania-based AmeriGas Propane waives copayments for prescription anti-smoking treatments and provides smokers with other incentives to quit. And Washington State–based Destination Harley Davidson, which in 2001 began offering access to smoking-cessation programs at no cost, has found that employees who stop smoking have improved productivity and take fewer sick days.

Be Prepared for Relapse or Difficult Situations

Step 5 is to be kind to yourself if you slip up. Most relapses occur within the first 3 months after quitting. Don't be discouraged if you start smoking again. Remember, most people try several times (on average, three) before they finally quit. The following are some difficult situations you may encounter:

◆ Alcohol. Avoid drinking alcohol. Drinking lowers your chances of success.

◆ Other smokers. Being around smoking can make you want to smoke.

◆ Weight gain. Many smokers will gain some weight when they quit, usually less than 10 pounds. Eat a healthy diet and stay active. Don't let weight gain distract you from your main goal—quitting smoking. Some quit-smoking medications may help delay weight gain.

◆ Bad mood or depression. There are a lot of ways to improve your mood other than smoking. Some quit-smoking medications also lessen depression.

If you are having problems with any of these situations, talk to your doctor or other health-care provider.

Special Situations or Conditions

Studies suggest that everyone can quit smoking. Your situation or condition can give you a special reason to quit.

◆ Pregnant women/new mothers. By quitting, you protect your baby's health and your own.

◆ Hospitalized patients. By quitting, you reduce health problems and help healing.

◆ Heart attack patients. By quitting, you reduce your risk of a second heart attack.

◆ Lung, head, and neck cancer patients. By quitting, you reduce your chance of a second cancer.

◆ Parents of children and adolescents. By quitting, you protect your children and adolescents from illnesses caused by secondhand smoke.

Questions to Think About

Think about the following questions before you try to stop smoking. You may want to talk about your answers with your health-care provider.

◆ Why do you want to quit?

◆ When you tried to quit in the past, what helped and what didn't?

◆ What will be the most difficult situations for you after you quit? How will you plan to handle them?

◆ Who can help you through the tough times? Your family? Friends? Health-care provider?

◆ What pleasures do you get from smoking? What ways can you still get pleasure if you quit?

Here are some questions to ask your health-care provider:

◆ How can you help me to be successful at quitting?

◆ What medication do you think would be best for me and how should I take it?

◆ What should I do if I need more help?

◆ What is smoking withdrawal like? How can I get information on withdrawal?

Getting Enough Shut-Eye

According to the National Institutes of Health, insomnia affects more than 70 million Americans. Insomnia is characterized by difficulty falling asleep, difficulty staying asleep, and waking too early in the morning.

Sleep loss can impair your memory, learning, logical reasoning, and physical coordination. A sleep disorder called sleep apnea can lead to high blood pressure, heart attack, and stroke.

InflamWise

People who have sleep apnea stop breathing for 10 to 30 seconds at a time while they are sleeping. It can be a dangerous sleep problem, and many people with the problem do not realize they have it.

According to the American Academy of Family Physicians, your risk of heart disease and stroke is higher if you have serious sleep apnea and you do not get treatment.

If you have sleep apnea or unexplained fatigue, it is very important for you to get treatment. The American Sleep Apnea Association offers assistance and support groups for people with sleep apnea. Their contact information is listed in Appendix B.

The amount of sleep each person needs to function properly and remain healthy varies. You may need 8 hours and your husband needs only 6. In general, most adults need approximately 7 to 9 hours of sleep a night.

What causes poor sleep?

◆ Stress—school or job pressures, family or marriage problems, serious illness or death

◆ Too much caffeine or alcohol, or exercising too close to your bedtime

- Jet lag

- Distracting sleep environment—too cold or hot, too bright, too noisy

- Some medications, including decongestants, steroids, and some medicines for high blood pressure, asthma, or depression

What Can I Do to Get a Good Night's Sleep?

Here are some tips for getting a restful night's sleep:

- Avoid stimulants such as caffeine, nicotine and alcohol before bedtime.

- Exercise regularly.

- Use your bed only for sleep or sexual activity.

- If you have trouble sleeping, don't nap during the day.

- Establish a regular bedtime routine that lets your brain know it's time to sleep.

- If you can't sleep, get up and do something relaxing, such as reading, to clear your mind.

If your sleep problem persists more than a week, and if your lack of sleep interferes with your ability to function during the day, consult a physician.

The Least You Need to Know

- Meditation can help you relax and improve health.

- Relaxed breathing can help you control your stress.

- The good news about smoking is that you can quit. Many people have done it successfully.

- Lack of sleep and sleep apnea can have serious health consequences. If a sleep problem lasts more than a week, see a doctor.

Chapter 17

Exercise and Weight Control

In This Chapter

- ◆ Learn how to measure activity levels
- ◆ See the advantages of strength training
- ◆ Walk your way to health
- ◆ Discover tips on how to get proper instruction
- ◆ Preventing injury

The evidence is clear. Regardless of your age, exercise improves health. It helps to control weight (preventing metabolic syndrome and inflammation in the process); contributes to a healthy heart, bones, muscles, and joints; reduces falls among older adults; helps people sleep better; helps to relieve the pain of arthritis; reduces symptoms of anxiety and depression; and is associated with fewer hospitalizations, physician visits, and medications.

Regular physical activity also reduces the risk of dying from coronary heart disease, stroke, colon cancer, diabetes, and high blood pressure.

This chapter covers tips on how to add activity and exercise into your daily life.

We Need to Get Moving!

Although it's clear that the benefits of exercise are endless, as a society we tend to be slackers.

Despite the proven benefits of physical activity:

◆ More than 50 percent of American adults do not get enough physical activity to provide health benefits.

◆ 25 percent of adults are not active at all in their leisure time.

Exercise and Children

Lack of exercise contributes greatly to the obesity epidemic among children. More than a third of young people in grades 9 through 12 do not regularly engage in vigorous-intensity physical activity. And children spend an average of 3 to 4 hours a day watching TV.

Exercise should start in childhood to promote improved cardiovascular health in adult life.

Developing a Plan

Physical activity need not be strenuous to be health-promoting and to help control weight, and people of all ages benefit from regular physical activity.

If you are a beginner, it is important to find the type of exercise that you will enjoy. Otherwise, it will be hard to stick to. It's also important to start out slowly and work your way up to a higher level of activity.

Measuring Activity

In order to gain the benefits of exercise, you should strive to meet either of the following physical activity recommendations:

◆ Engage in moderate-intensity physical activities for at least 30 minutes on 5 or more days of the week.

Moderate-intensity physical activity means that your breathing or heart rate speeds up during exercise.

◆ Engage in vigorous-intensity (*aerobic*) physical activity 3 or more days per week for 20 or more minutes per occasion.

def•i•ni•tion

Aerobic activity is brisk physical activity that requires the heart and lungs to work harder to meet the body's increased oxygen demand. Aerobic exercise promotes the circulation of oxygen through the blood and improves cardiovascular fitness.

Vigorous-intensity physical activity is intense enough to represent a substantial challenge while exercising. It refers to a level of effort in which you have a large increase in breathing or heart rate.

Another measure of activity level is how many calories you burn as you exercise. The chart below shows the approximate calories spent per hour by a 150-pound person doing a particular activity.

> **Did You Know?**
>
> Walking up stairs burns almost five times more calories than riding an elevator.

Physical Activity Calorie Use Chart

Activity for 150 lb. Person	Calories
Bicycling, 6 mph	240
Bicycling, 12 mph	410
Jogging, 7 mph	780
Swimming, 25 yds/min	275
Swimming, 50 yds/min	500
Tennis singles	400
Walking, 2 mph	240
Walking, 3 mph	320
Walking, 4.5 mph	440

The Talk Test

The "talk test" method of measuring intensity is simple. If you are active at a light intensity level you should be able to sing while doing the activity. If you are active at a moderate intensity level, you should be able to carry on a conversation comfortably while engaging in the activity. If you become too winded or too out of breath to carry on a conversation, the activity is vigorous.

InflamWise

Physical activity is a lot more fun if you do it with a buddy. Most of us agree that the hardest thing about getting exercise is staying motivated. An exercise buddy can make it twice as fun. For example, arrange to meet a friend three times a week for a vigorous walk and a good chat! Or go to a dance class with a partner, or arrange to join friends for golf or tennis. There is something magical about making a date for exercise—most of us are far more likely to not put it off and to show up.

Activities and Their Intensity Levels

Higher-intensity activities require less time spent to gain the cardiac and other benefits. Lower-intensity activities require more time spent.

Levels of Activity

Light-Intensity Activities:

- Walking slowly
- Golf, powered cart
- Swimming, slow treading
- Gardening or pruning
- Bicycling, very light effort
- Dusting or vacuuming
- Conditioning exercise, light stretching, or warm-up

Moderate-Intensity Activities

- Walking briskly
- Golf, pulling or carrying clubs
- Swimming, recreational
- Mowing lawn, power motor

- Tennis, doubles

- Bicycling 5 to 9 mph, level terrain, or with a few hills

- Scrubbing floors or washing windows

- Weight lifting, Nautilus machines or free weights

Vigorous-Intensity Activities:

- Racewalking, jogging, or running

- Swimming laps

- Mowing lawn, hand mower

- Tennis, singles

- Bicycling more than 10 mph, or on steep uphill terrain

- Moving or pushing furniture

- Circuit training

If you have a chronic disease, such as a heart condition, arthritis, diabetes, or high blood pressure, you should talk to your doctor about what types and amounts of physical activity are appropriate.

If you have symptoms that could be due to a chronic disease, you should have these symptoms checked, whether you are active or inactive. If you plan to start a new activity program, take the opportunity to get these symptoms evaluated.

Symptoms of particular importance to evaluate include chest pain (especially chest pain that is brought on by exertion), loss of balance (especially loss of balance leading to a fall), dizziness, and passing out (loss of consciousness).

How to Avoid Injury

The most common risk associated with physical activity is injury to your bones, joints, tendons, and muscles.

If you are a beginner, you should start out slowly to prevent soreness and injury. This way you will gradually build up to the desired amount of activity and give your body time to adjust.

Getting Instruction

Injury can occur because of making incorrect movements while exercising. It happens even to seasoned athletes. Getting instruction can cut down on this type of injury, and the social interaction with an instructor or in a class can make getting exercise more fun. Here are some tips:

◆ Take a class. A knowledgeable group fitness instructor will be able to teach you how to exercise with proper form and lower the risk of injury. The instructor can watch your actions during class and let you know if you are doing things right. You can also mimic the instructor's movements, making it easier to learn how to do specific exercises.

◆ Try water workouts. Whether you swim laps or take water aerobics, working out in the water is easy on your joints and helps reduce sore muscles and injury. Warm water is great for sore joints.

◆ Work with a personal trainer. A certified personal trainer will be able to show you how to warm up, cool down, use fitness equipment like treadmills and weight-training machines, and use proper form to help lower your risk for injury.

◆ Check out your local health, recreation, or community center.

◆ Join or start a walking, jogging, or biking group. You can enjoy added safety and company as you walk.

Preventing Injury

Keeping the following tips in mind can help prevent common injuries during exercise:

◆ Use appropriate equipment and clothing for the activity.

◆ Take 3 to 5 minutes at the beginning of any physical activity to properly warm up your muscles through increasingly more intense activity.

◆ As you near the end of the activity, cool down by decreasing the level of intensity. For example, before jogging, walk for 3 to 5 minutes, increasing your pace to a brisk walk. After jogging, walk briskly, decreasing your pace to a slow walk over 3 to 5 minutes. Finish by stretching the muscles you used—in this case primarily the muscles of the legs.

◆ Start at an easy pace, increasing time or distance gradually.

◆ Drink plenty of water throughout the day to replace lost fluids. Drink a glass of water before you start your exercise, and drink another half cup every 15 minutes that you remain active.

Stretching

Stretching is important to keep your muscles from getting tight and to increase flexibility. It may also help keep you limber. Do stretching exercises after endurance and strength training, when your muscles are warm.

It is best to learn how to stretch from a qualified trainer to make sure that you are doing it correctly. Always get your blood flowing and body warmed before you stretch.

Strength Training

There are numerous benefits to strength training, particularly as you grow older. Hippocrates explained the principle behind strength training when he wrote "that which is used develops, and that which is not used wastes away."

Strength training is a form of exercise in which you develop the strength and size of the muscles that support your bones. Properly performed, strength training can help you move around and carry out tasks better. This type of training is not the same thing as bodybuilding, weightlifting, and powerlifting, which are sports.

The following sections include facts from a report by the Centers for Disease Control and Prevention about the benefits of strength training.

Arthritis Relief

Tufts University recently conducted a strength-training program with older men and women with moderate to severe osteoarthritis of the knee. The results of this 16-week program showed that strength training decreased pain by 43 percent, increased muscle strength and general physical performance, improved the clinical signs and symptoms of the disease, and decreased disability.

Here is the important point: the effectiveness of strength training to ease the pain of osteoarthritis was just as potent, if not more potent, as medications. Similar effects of strength training have been seen in patients with rheumatoid arthritis.

Restoration of Balance and Reduction of Falls

Poor balance and flexibility contribute to falls and broken bones. These fractures can result in significant disability and, in some cases, death. One study in New Zealand in women 80 years of age and older showed a 40 percent reduction in falls with simple strength and balance training.

Strengthening of Bone

After menopause women can lose 1 to 2 percent of their bone mass annually. Results from a study conducted at Tufts University showed that strength training increases bone density and reduces the risk for fractures among women aged 50 to 70.

Proper Weight Maintenance

Strength training is crucial to weight control because individuals who have more muscle mass have a high rate of metabolism. Strength training can provide up to a 15 percent increase in metabolism.

Improved Glucose Control

Studies show that lifestyle changes such as strength training can help people who have diabetes. In a recent study of Hispanic men and women, 16 weeks of strength training produced dramatic improvements in glucose control, comparable to taking diabetes medication. Additionally, the study volunteers were stronger, gained muscle, lost body fat, had less depression, and felt much more self-confident.

Pump!

Lifting weights is the most common method of strength training. Most gyms have weights, and weights are readily available for purchase in most sports and department stores.

With this technique, you exercise all your major muscle groups at least twice a week. However, it is important not to exercise the same muscle group two days in a row. If you are a beginner, be sure to get instruction on the proper way to lift weights.

InflamWise

Many people wonder what equipment they should buy to start weight training. A complete workout can be performed with a pair of adjustable dumbbells (or barbells) and a set of weight disks (plates). (Dumbbells and barbells are weights that are not attached to anything and are raised and lowered using your hands and arms.) Most local sports or big-box stores carry them. They should be affordable—there is no reason to spend a lot of money on them.

Here are some guidelines from the National Institutes of Health:

◆ Gradually increasing the amount of weight you use is the most important part of strength exercise.

◆ Start with a low amount of weight (or no weight) and increase it gradually.

◆ When you are ready to progress, first increase the number of times you do the exercise, then increase the weight at a later session.

◆ Do an exercise 8 to 15 times; rest a minute and repeat it 8 to 15 more times.

◆ Take 3 seconds to lift and 3 seconds to lower weights. Never jerk weights into position.

◆ If you can't lift a weight more than eight times, it's too heavy; if you can lift it more than 15 times, it's too light.

◆ Avoid holding your breath while straining.

◆ Weight training may make you sore at first, but it should never cause pain.

◆ Stretch after strength-building exercises.

Resistance Bands

Resistance bands are giant rubber bands that you pull against (resist) to strengthen certain muscle groups. Resistance bands are more convenient than most weight-lifting gear, and they're inexpensive. They are also portable; you can take them with you when you travel. (So no excuses!)

An example of an exercise with resistance bands is to place the end of the band under your feet while standing, hold the other end in one or both hands, and pull up against the band.

Another exercise is to use a band with handles on either end and hold it by the feet while seated on the ground with legs outstretched. Taking a handle in either hand, pull with both back and shoulder muscles to work the same muscle groups that a rowing machine would exercise.

As always, however, it is important to learn these and other movements from an exercise professional.

Resistance bands come in different levels, from easy-to-stretch to progressively more difficult. If you're a beginner, start at the lowest level of resistance and work your way to higher levels.

Pilates

Pilates is an increasingly popular exercise program based on building core strength. Pilates teaches body awareness, good posture, and easy, graceful movement. The program emphasizes proper breathing, correct spinal and pelvic alignment, and complete concentration on smooth, flowing movement.

Through this method you become acutely aware of how your body feels, where it is in space, and how to control its movement. Proper breathing is essential in Pilates. Learning to breathe properly greatly reduces stress.

Pilates classes take place with machines called "reformers" or on floor mats. Many instructional video programs are available, but if you are a beginner it is important to start by getting instruction from a well-trained professional. Learning to do the exercises correctly is important to prevent injury and get the full benefits of the program.

Walking Your Way to Health

Experts stress that if you do no other exercise, at the very least get out and walk for health. With the exception of the cost of a comfortable shoe with good support, walking is free, simple, and convenient. It can help you control your weight (and prevent metabolic syndrome). And it is one of the best things you can do for your heart.

Walking and Weight Control

Walking 1 mile can burn up at least 100 calories of energy; walking 2 miles a day, three times a week, can help reduce weight by 1 pound every 3 weeks. Walking also alters fat metabolism so that fat is burned up instead of sugars, helping to reduce weight and prevent metabolic syndrome.

Get More Out of Your Walk

For many of us, brisk walking for 30 minutes most days of the week is a great way to get aerobic exercise. Brisk walking requires the heart and lungs to work harder to meet the body's increased oxygen demand.

Try these techniques for getting the most out of your walking program:

◆ Walking with extra weight increases the aerobic benefit. Be sure to distribute weight evenly across your body. Belts or vests with pockets for inserting weights work the best.

◆ Most exercise experts do not recommend strapping exercise weights around the ankle or wrists when walking because they can strain muscles.

InflamWise

Walking is the best possible exercise. Habituate yourself to walk very far.

—Thomas Jefferson, 3rd President of the United States

◆ As you walk, contract your stomach muscles often.

◆ Make sure you are walking up a hill part of the time.

◆ Use resistance bands with your arms as you walk. Pull and stretch them using your major muscle groups.

Signs of Overdoing It

It is important to start slowly and not overdo it when you start a walking program. You may want to walk only 15 minutes the first day, then increase to 20 minutes for a few days, and so on.

If you experience any of the following signs, you have been overly zealous:

◆ You are too worn out to finish. You should be able to finish with energy to spare.

◆ You cannot carry on a normal conversation while walking.

◆ You feel faint or nauseous after walking.

◆ You are worn out for the rest of the day.

◆ You experience increased aches and pains. You will feel some discomfort in your muscles due to increased activity. However, your joints should not hurt and you should not be stiff. Make sure to warm up and stretch.

When It's Serious

Make sure that you know the symptoms that, if they occur while walking or during any other type of exercise, can signal a serious health problem. Check with your doctor or other health-care provider before exercising again if any of these signs occur:

◆ Pain or discomfort in the chest, arm, upper body, neck, or jaw

◆ Faintness or lightheadedness

◆ Shortness of breath

◆ Irregular pulse

◆ Changes in normal symptoms such as the amount of chest pain or increased joint pain

In addition to walking, biking is an easy, inexpensive, and convenient way to get exercise.

Bicycling

Riding a bicycle is great exercise, and it is easier on your joints than running or jogging. Make sure that you are riding safely. Here are some tips:

◆ To avoid injury to your head and face, wear a helmet even on short trips. Make sure your helmet meets government standards. Helmets are now required in some states.

◆ Wearing a pair of sport sunglasses can stop dust from getting in your eyes.

◆ Wear bright, reflective clothing so that drivers see you. Make sure that you have reflectors on your bike.

◆ Wear lights at night.

◆ Wear padded gloves to protect your hands.

◆ Wear padded shorts and use a comfortable seat to reduce buttock pain.

◆ Parents should teach children basic traffic rules and make sure they ride in safe places.

◆ Children younger than 10 should not ride near traffic.

◆ Be extremely careful in traffic. You could be seriously hurt if you run into a car or if you are riding fast. Children can be hurt while doing stunts on their bicycles.

◆ Make sure that everything on your bicycle is in working order. Check your brakes regularly; make sure there are no loose or broken parts on your bike.

◆ If you ride with a child on your bicycle, use a special seat that fits behind the main seat. You and your child both need to wear helmets. Make sure the bike has spoke guards to prevent the child's feet from getting caught in the spokes.

> **What the Experts Say**
>
> *The bicycle is the most efficient machine ever created: Converting calories into gas, a bicycle gets the equivalent of three thousand miles per gallon.*
>
> —Bill Strickland, *The Quotable Cyclist*, Breakaway Books, 1997

Fitting Physical Activity into Your Daily Life

Are you stumped on how to fit physical activity into your life? Listed below are several suggestions for any time of day.

At Home

Here are some tips to fit exercise into your routine at home:

◆ Make physical activity a priority. Make time each week to be active and put it on your calendar. Try waking up a half-hour earlier to walk, or take an evening fitness class.

◆ Build physical activity into your routine chores. Rake the yard, wash the car, and do energetic housework.

◆ Make family time physically active. Plan a weekend hike through a park, a family softball game, or an evening walk around the block.

◆ Many people combine exercise with other activities, such as watching TV or listening to audiobooks. Try walking in place while watching TV.

◆ Exercise equipment is a one-time expense and other family members can use it. Find used equipment in the classifieds.

◆ Keep exercise equipment repaired and use it!

◆ Do your own house and yard work.

◆ Walk the dog. If you don't have a dog, walk your neighbor's dog.

◆ When you go shopping, park far away from the building and walk the extra distance.

◆ Stretch to reach items in high places and squat or bend to look at items at floor level.

◆ Meet a friend for workouts. If your friend is on the next bike or treadmill, you will enjoy it more.

◆ Get outside. A change in scenery can relieve your boredom. If you are riding a bike, rollerblading, or skateboarding, be sure to wear a helmet.

At Work

One of the most difficult places to fit in exercise is at the office. But some simple tips can help you add physical activity to your work day:

◆ Take frequent walks around the office. Have "walk and talk meetings."

◆ Stand and stretch when talking on the telephone.

◆ Take the stairs instead of the elevator.

◆ Start an exercise class at your company. You and your colleagues could chip in for an instructor to come in during the lunch hour.

◆ Form a walk or run team to raise money for charity events.

◆ Join a fitness center near your job. Exercise before or after work to avoid rush-hour traffic.

◆ Walk around your building for a break during the workday or during lunch.

On the Road

Traveling can get in the way of getting adequate exercise. Here are some tips for fitting exercise into your trips away from home:

◆ Walk around the concourse at the airport while waiting for a plane.

 ◆ Take exercise clothes with you and stay at hotels with fitness centers or swimming pools.

 ◆ Take a jump rope, stretch bands, and other packable equipment when you travel.

 ◆ Jump and do calisthenics in your hotel room.

 ◆ If it's safe, get outdoors and walk around the area where you are staying.

At Play

Building physical activity into your playtime has a double benefit: you can get exercise while having fun.

 ◆ Look for opportunities to be active and have fun at the same time.

 ◆ Plan outings and vacations with family and friends that include physical activity (hiking, backpacking, swimming, etc.)

 ◆ Make a date with friends to play tennis, take a run, or hike.

 ◆ Take dancing lessons. Then, dance!

 ◆ Join a recreational club.

 ◆ When golfing, walk instead of using a cart.

The Least You Need to Know

 ◆ Do a moderate-intensity physical activity for at least 30 minutes on 5 or more days of the week.

 ◆ Or do a vigorous-intensity physical activity 3 or more days per week for 20 or more minutes per occasion.

 ◆ Do strength training regularly.

 ◆ Have a good instructor show you the proper way to use resistance bands and conduct other exercises.

 ◆ Walk or bicycle for health.

Part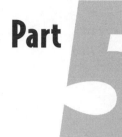

Anti-Inflammation Cooking

The final chapter of this book gives you the lowdown on popular and special diets and how they fit into your anti-inflammation way of life. We give a green light to three popular diets and offer our opinions about others. You will also find tips and recipes to try if you are on a low-salt, gluten-free, or lactose-free diet.

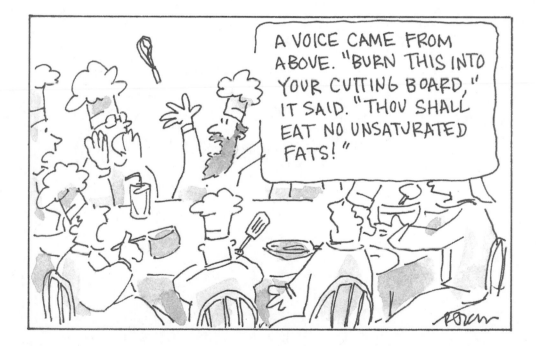

18

Special and Popular Diets

In This Chapter

- ◆ Learn about some major weight-loss diets
- ◆ Understand the DASH eating plan
- ◆ Discover tips for the wheat-free kitchen
- ◆ Discover tips for the dairy-free kitchen

If you're diabetic, have a heart condition, or are trying to lose weight, there's a good chance that you are on a special diet, which can create challenges for staying with the anti-inflammation plan. To help guide you, this chapter describes weight-loss and special-needs diets and how they can fit into your anti-inflammation lifestyle.

Weight-Loss Diets

Here is the bottom line: when following a weight-loss diet, make sure that it's compatible with the seven principles of the anti-inflammation diet. Here are details on some of the most popular weight-loss diets.

Only three popular diets get our green light, which means that they fit well with our anti-inflammatory diet plan. They are the South Beach Diet; the

Eat, Drink, and Weigh Less Diet; and Weight Watchers. Here are quick descriptions of them:

The South Beach Diet

The South Beach Diet, developed by Dr. Arthur Agatston, touts an eating plan of "good" carbohydrates (whole grains, fruits, and vegetables) and "good" fats (unsaturated). The premise is that you eat foods that it takes your body longer to absorb. It eliminates highly processed foods, saturated fats, and sugar, all to the good. We give it a green light.

Eat, Drink, and Weigh Less

This diet, by Dr. Walter C. Willet and Mollie Katzen, features the "Body Score" as a way to chart your progress. The more you raise your Body Score, the more you lower your weight. The book explaining the diet includes a quiz to help readers determine their Body Score; the chapters that follow explain easy dietary and behavioral steps individuals can take to improve their scores.

This diet is based on years of top research conducted by Willett, the head of Harvard Medical School of Public Health's Department of Nutrition, including the famous Nurses' Health Study. The study scored each of its over 84,000 participants on food choices, exercise schedule, and body mass—resulting in a number that accurately determined the nurses' risk of heart disease. It gets a green light.

Weight Watchers Winning Points System

This popular system assigns point values to different foods based on their nutritional content. Each day you have a certain range of points that you must stay within based on your current weight. If you follow the guidelines, you lose weight. The point system is based on examining calories, fat, and fiber. Fat increases point value; fiber decreases it. Most vegetables have no points or are low in points. Foods with high point values include sweets, pasta, rice, bread, and potatoes.

This system is easy to follow and is nutritionally balanced. It takes some work, but it is possible to stay on the anti-inflammation diet and this plan at the same time.

Other Popular Diets

In this section, we have included brief comments on other popular diets.

The Zone

The Zone Diet, developed by Dr. Barry Sears, emphasizes a ratio of carbohydrates (40 percent), fat (30 percent), and proteins (30 percent). It promotes weight loss by keeping insulin levels within "The Zone." Eating the right ratio lowers insulin levels, resulting in a metabolic state that increases energy and decreases hunger.

The Zone Diet focuses on lean proteins combined with vegetables, fruits, and healthy fats. A small amount of starchy carbohydrates can also be included in meals. Anything made with white flour, white sugar, and/or saturated fats is avoided. The safety of this diet has not been determined.

The Pritikin Diet

The Pritikin Diet, developed by Robert Pritikin, claims that cutting calorie density is the key to weight loss. The Pritikin Diet advocates fruits, vegetables, pasta, oatmeal, soups, salads, low-fat dairy; limited amounts of low-fat poultry, seafood, and meat; few fatty foods; and a limited amount of dry foods (crackers, popcorn, pretzels, and so on). This diet restricts seafood and low-fat poultry and is low in calcium, iron, zinc, vitamin D, vitamin E, and vitamin B12.

The Ornish Diet (Eat More, Weigh Less)

This diet was developed by Dr. Dean Ornish. Its premise is that if you eat fat-free, healthy foods, you can feel full and still lose weight. The diet includes vegetables, fruits, whole grains, beans, limited nonfat dairy (yogurt, cottage cheese), and egg whites. The diet emphasizes high levels of healthy carbohydrates (whole grains, fruits, and vegetables), no refined products, very low levels of fat, and about 15 percent protein. Many people feel this diet is too stringent to follow. It also restricts seafood, which we require for omega-3 fatty acids, and is deficient in zinc and vitamin B12.

The Atkins Diet

This famous diet, by Dr. Robert Atkins, restricts carbohydrates. The Atkins Diet recommends that you take in 50 to 55 percent of your total calories from fat, 30 to 40 percent of your calories from protein, and 5 to 15 percent of your calories from carbohydrates. This diet does not fit within our guidelines, but may have some value because people do lose weight on it, which is beneficial to prevent metabolic syndrome.

The Eat Right for Your Type Diet

This diet, developed by Dr. Peter D'Adamo, purports that diets should be individualized for people with different blood types. It is similar to the Atkins Diet.

The GI (Glycemic Index) Diet

The Glycemic Index Diet focuses on eating foods with a low glycemic index (GI) value, which leads to a metabolic state in which the body feels full longer, has increased energy, and experiences decreased hunger. The Glycemic Index Diet allows for three meals a day plus several snacks. It cuts risk factors for heart disease and diabetes better than conventional low-fat diets. This diet has promise, but it is too complicated for most people to follow.

The Sonoma Diet

The Sonoma Diet was developed by Connie Guttersen, a dietitian at the Culinary Institute of America in St. Helena, California. The diet follows the principles of the Mediterranean region, with an emphasis on healthful fats, fish, nuts, lean meats, and whole grains. And it cuts back on white flour.

Diets for Special Needs

The following sections include information on special diets, including the DASH Eating Plan for Hypertension, the American Heart Association Eating Plan, the American Diabetes Association Meal Plan, the Dairy-Free Kitchen, and the Wheat-Free Kitchen.

The DASH Eating Plan for Hypertension

The DASH Eating Plan for Hypertension is a diet based on two studies supported by the National Heart, Lung, and Blood Institute (NHLBI). Its results showed that blood pressures were reduced with an eating plan that is low in saturated fat, cholesterol, and total fat, and that emphasizes fruits, vegetables, and low-fat dairy foods. This eating plan—known as the DASH eating plan—also includes whole-grain products, fish, poultry, and nuts. It is reduced in red meat, sweets, and sugar-containing beverages. It is rich in magnesium, potassium, and calcium, as well as protein and fiber.

In the first study by the NHLBI, DASH compared three eating plans: a plan similar in nutrients to what many Americans consume, a plan similar to what Americans consume but higher in fruits and vegetables, and the DASH eating plan. All three plans included about 3,000 milligrams of sodium daily. None of the plans was vegetarian or used specialty foods.

Results were dramatic: both the fruits and vegetables plan and the DASH eating plan reduced blood pressure. But the DASH eating plan had the greatest effect, especially for those with high blood pressure. Furthermore, the blood pressure reductions came fast—within 2 weeks of starting the plan.

The second study was called "DASH-Sodium," and it looked at the effect on blood pressure of a reduced dietary sodium intake as participants followed either the DASH eating plan or an eating plan typical of what many Americans consume.

Participants were randomly assigned to one of the two eating plans and then followed for a month at each of three sodium levels. The three sodium levels were a higher intake of about 3,300 milligrams per day (the level consumed by many Americans); an intermediate intake of about 2,400 milligrams per day; and a lower intake of about 1,500 milligrams per day.

Results showed that reducing dietary sodium lowered blood pressure for both eating plans. At each sodium level, blood pressure was lower on the DASH eating plan than on the other eating plan.

The biggest blood pressure reductions were for the DASH eating plan at the sodium intake of 1,500 milligrams per day. Those with hypertension saw the biggest reductions, but those without it also had large decreases.

Those on the 1,500-milligram sodium intake eating plan, as well as those on the DASH eating plan, had fewer headaches. Other than that and blood pressure levels, there were no significant effects caused by the two eating plans or different sodium levels.

The DASH-Sodium study shows the importance of lowering sodium intake—regardless of what you eat.

This DASH sample plan is based on 2,000 calories a day.

◆ Grains and grain products: 7 to 8 servings, 1 slice bread, ½ cup cooked rice

◆ Vegetables: 4 to 5 servings: 1 cup raw leafy, ½ cup cooked vegetable peas, 6 oz. vegetable juice

◆ Fruits: 4 to 5 servings, 6 oz. fruit juice, 1 medium fruit, $^1/_2$ cup fresh, frozen, or canned fruit

◆ Low-fat or fat-free dairy foods: 2 to 3 servings, 8 oz. milk, 1 cup yogurt, $1^1/_2$ oz. cheese

◆ Meats, poultry, and fish: 2 or less, 3 oz. cooked meats, poultry, or fish

◆ Nuts, seeds, and dry beans: 4 to 5 servings per week, $^1/_3$ cup or $1^1/_2$ oz. nuts, 2 TB. or $^1/_2$ oz. seeds, $^1/_2$ cup cooked dry beans, peas

◆ Fats and oils: 2 to 3 servings, 1 tsp. soft margarine, 1 TB. low-fat mayonnaise, 2 TB. light salad dressing, 1 tsp. vegetable oil (DASH has 27 percent of calories from fat)

◆ Sweets: 5 per week, 1 TB. sugar, 1 TB. jam or jelly, $^1/_2$ oz. jelly beans, 8 oz. lemonade (sweets should be low in fat)

DASH Tips to Reduce Salt and Sodium

The DASH plan includes excellent tips for anyone who needs to reduce their salt intake:

◆ Use reduced-sodium or no-salt-added products. For example, choose low- or reduced-sodium, or no-salt-added versions of foods and condiments when available.

◆ Buy fresh, frozen, or canned with no-salt-added vegetables.

◆ Use fresh poultry, fish, and lean meat, rather than canned, smoked, or processed types.

◆ Choose ready-to-eat breakfast cereals that are lower in sodium.

◆ Limit cured foods (such as bacon and ham), foods packed in brine (such as pickles, pickled vegetables, olives, and sauerkraut), and condiments (such as MSG, mustard, horseradish, catsup, and barbecue sauce). Limit even lower-sodium versions of soy sauce and teriyaki sauce—treat these condiments as you do table salt.

◆ Use spices instead of salt. In cooking and at the table, flavor foods with herbs, spices, lemon, lime, vinegar, or salt-free seasoning blends. Start by cutting salt in half.

◆ Cook rice, pasta, and hot cereals without salt. Cut back on instant or flavored rice, pasta, and cereal mixes, which usually have added salt.

◆ Choose "convenience" foods that are lower in sodium. Cut back on frozen dinners, mixed dishes such as pizza, packaged mixes, canned soups or broths, and salad dressings—these often have a lot of sodium.

◆ Rinse canned foods, such as tuna, to remove some sodium.

Controlling Sodium When Eating Out

Here are some tips for cutting back on sodium when eating in restaurants.

◆ Ask how foods are prepared. Ask that they be prepared without added salt, MSG, or salt-containing ingredients. Most restaurants are willing to accommodate requests.

◆ Know the terms that indicate high sodium content: pickled, cured, soy sauce, broth.

◆ Move the salt shaker away.

◆ Limit condiments, such as mustard, ketchup, pickles, and sauces with salt-containing ingredients.

◆ Choose fruits or vegetables instead of salty snack foods.

When Shopping

The following is a list of the words that you will run into to describe sodium content, and what those words actually mean:

◆ Sodium-free or salt-free: Less than 5 milligrams per serving.

◆ Very low sodium: 35 milligrams or less of sodium per serving.

◆ Low sodium: 140 milligrams or less of sodium per serving.

◆ Low-sodium meal: 140 milligrams or less of sodium per $3\frac{1}{2}$ ounces (100 grams).

◆ Reduced or less sodium: At least 25 percent less sodium than the regular version.

◆ Light in sodium: 50 percent less sodium than the regular version.

◆ Unsalted or no salt added: No salt added to the product during processing.

The American Heart Association

The American Heart Association Eating Plan for Healthy Americans is based on reducing three of the major risk factors for heart attack—high blood cholesterol, high blood pressure, and excess body weight. Here are some of the guidelines:

◆ Eat a variety of fruits and vegetables. Choose five or more servings per day.

◆ Eat a variety of grain products, including whole grains. Choose six or more servings per day.

◆ Include fat-free and low-fat milk products, fish, legumes (beans), skinless poultry, and lean meats.

◆ Choose fats and oils with 2 grams or less saturated fat per tablespoon, such as liquid and tub margarines, canola oil, and olive oil.

◆ Balance the number of calories you eat with the number you use each day.

◆ Maintain a level of physical activity that keeps you fit and matches the number of calories you eat. Walk or do other activities for at least 30 minutes on most days.

◆ To lose weight, do enough activity to use up more calories than you eat every day.

◆ Limit your intake of foods high in calories or low in nutrition, including foods like soft drinks and candy that have a lot of sugars.

◆ Limit foods high in saturated fat, trans fat, and/or cholesterol, such as full-fat milk products, fatty meats, tropical oils, partially hydrogenated vegetable oils, and egg yolks. Eat less than 6 grams of salt (sodium chloride) per day (2,400 milligrams of sodium).

Have no more than one alcoholic drink per day if you're a woman and no more than two if you're a man. "One drink" means it has no more than $1/2$ ounce of pure alcohol. Examples of one drink are 12 ounces of beer, 4 ounces of wine, $1 1/2$ ounces of 80-proof spirits, or 1 ounce of 100-proof spirits.

The American Diabetes Association (ADA) Meal Plan

The ADA meal plan tells you how much and what kinds of food you can choose to eat at meals and snack times. People with diabetes have to take extra care to make sure that their food is balanced with insulin and oral medications, and exercise to help manage their blood glucose levels. The approach involves working with your doctor and/or dietitian to create a meal plan that works for you.

The Dairy-Free Kitchen

Lactose intolerance is the inability to digest significant amounts of lactose, the major sugar found in dairy products. It is caused by a shortage of the enzyme lactase, which is produced by the cells that line the small intestine. Lactose intolerance is sometimes the result of inflammation in the intestine.

What are the symptoms of lactose intolerance?

People who do not have enough lactase to digest the amount of lactose they consume may feel very uncomfortable when they digest milk products. Common symptoms, which range from mild to severe, include nausea, cramps, bloating, gas, and diarrhea. Symptoms begin about 30 minutes to 2 hours after eating or drinking foods containing lactose.

There are medical tests that you can have taken to determine if you are lactose intolerance. If you suspect that you have the problem ask your doctor or other health-care provider about them.

What is hidden lactose?

Lactose is often added to prepared foods. People with very low tolerance for lactose should stay away from foods that may contain even small amounts of lactose, such as:

- ◆ Bread and other baked goods
- ◆ Processed breakfast cereals
- ◆ Instant potatoes, soups, and breakfast drinks
- ◆ Margarine
- ◆ Lunch meats (other than kosher)
- ◆ Salad dressings
- ◆ Candies and other snacks
- ◆ Mixes for pancakes, biscuits, and cookies
- ◆ Powdered meal-replacement supplements

Some products labeled nondairy, such as powdered coffee creamer and whipped toppings, may actually include ingredients that are derived from milk and therefore contain lactose.

People with lactose intolerance must read food labels with care, looking not only for milk and lactose, but also for words such as "whey," "curds," "milk by-products," "dry milk solids," and "nonfat dry milk powder." If any of these words are listed on a label, the product contains lactose.

Lactose is also used in more than 20 percent of prescription drugs and about 6 percent of over-the-counter medicines. Many types of birth control pills contain lactose, as do some tablets for stomach acid and gas. However, these products typically affect only people with severe lactose intolerance.

Many people with lactose intolerance can enjoy dairy products if they eat them in small amounts or eat other food at the same time. Lactase liquids or tablets are available to help with digestion. If you must limit dairy foods you can meet your need for calcium by eating greens, fish, and other calcium-rich foods that are free of lactose.

The Wheat-Free Kitchen

Gluten intolerance (celiac disease) is a genetic disorder that causes an allergy to a protein called gluten in wheat. This response leads to inflammation in the intestines and to the damage and destruction of cells in the lining of the intestinal wall.

> **Did You Know?**
>
> Although celiac disease can affect anyone, it tends to be more common in people of European descent and people with disorders caused by a reaction of the immune system (autoimmune disorders), such as lupus erythematosus, Type I diabetes, rheumatoid arthritis, and autoimmune thyroid disease.

Symptoms of gluten intolerance can include diarrhea, weight loss, malnutrition, mild weakness, bone pain, stomach swelling, and nutrient deficiencies. The most common foods that contain gluten are wheat, rye, and barley. Until recently it was thought that oats were a problem for people suffering from celiac disease. However, recent studies have shed doubt on this theory.

When people who are gluten intolerant continue consuming gluten, their chances of developing gastrointestinal cancer increase dramatically. Apart from this, their quality of life may be seriously undermined.

There are medical tests that you can have performed to determine if you have gluten intolerance. If you suspect that you have the problem, ask your doctor or other health provider.

People who are gluten intolerant must avoid foods with wheat for the rest of their life. This is sometimes a difficult task. Many products have hidden gluten in them. Watch out for any products that contain:

◆ Starch; many are wheat-based

◆ HVP (Hydrolyzed Vegetable Protein)

◆ HPP (Hydrolyzed Plant Protein)

◆ Maltodextrin; some are derived from wheat

◆ Wheat malt extract

◆ Malt vinegar

◆ Soy sauce; check to see if it is wheat-based

◆ Caramel coloring

Gluten- and Lactose-Free Recipes

The following recipes can add zest to a sodium-free diet.

Gluten-Free Taco Quesadillas

Do not use low-fat or fat-free sour cream with these quesadillas. They may contain gluten from maltodextrin and/or modified food starch.

2 TB. olive oil	4 soft corn tortillas
1 small onion, minced	1 cup shredded cheddar cheese
1 clove garlic, minced	
1 lb. ground turkey	½ head iceberg lettuce
2 tsp. cumin	2 large plum tomatoes, finely diced (1 cup)
2 tsp. chili powder	
1 tsp. salt	Chopped cilantro leaves, for garnish
1 tsp. black pepper	

Place oil in a skillet and sauté onions and garlic. Add turkey and brown. Drain fat and return to the pan. Add cumin, chili powder, salt, and pepper, mix thoroughly, and cook 1 to 2 minutes. Set aside.

Lay out tortillas and scatter cheese, meat mixture, lettuce, and tomatoes evenly over each.

Spray cooking spray on a skillet or grill pan. Heat pan. Fold filled tortillas in half, press down lightly and place on preheated grill pan. Cook 1 to 2 minutes, being careful tortillas do not burn. Flip tortillas carefully and grill an additional 1 to 2 minutes. Remove from heat and let cool a few minutes. Serve immediately. Serve with cilantro and corn salsa (next recipe).

Corn Salsa

4 ears yellow corn, roasted	1 TB. fresh lime juice
3 TB. olive oil	1 TB. fresh cilantro
1 large red tomato	½ tsp. salt
1 small jalapeño pepper	1 tsp. black pepper
1 garlic clove	⅛ tsp. ground cumin
2 TB. diced red pepper	

In medium bowl, combine all ingredients. Cover and refrigerate. Bring to room temperature before using.

Chicken Mole

2 TB. olive oil

4 lb. chicken parts with skin off

1 small onion

1 clove garlic

24 oz. homemade or store-purchased salsa

1 cup fat-free chicken broth

1 cup chili powder

3 TB. natural peanut butter

2 tsp. baking cocoa

8 cups cooked brown rice

½ cup chopped parsley

Heat oil in large skillet over medium-high heat. Add chicken; cook, turning frequently, for 4 to 6 minutes or until browned on all sides. Remove from skillet. Add onion and garlic; cook, stirring constantly, for 2 to 3 minutes or until onion is tender.

Stir in salsa, broth, chili powder, peanut butter, and cocoa. Bring to a boil. Reduce heat to medium-low. Add chicken; cook for 20 to 25 minutes or until chicken is no longer pink near bones. Mix brown rice and parsley. Serve with rice.

Baba Ganoush

2 large eggplants

¼ cup tahina

1 small onion

3–7 cloves of garlic

½–1 TB. cumin

1 tsp. ground coriander

1 tsp. vinegar

1–2 TB. lemon juice

1 TB. olive oil

Salt

Red pepper (optional)

Water

Pierce the skin of the eggplants (unless you want an exploding food episode!) and place on tinfoil under broiler.

Broil, turning once, until they are oozing and the skin is black on both sides. Throw the eggplants in cold water and peel. Drain the flesh and pop into a blender. Mix remaining ingredients and add a small amount; blend on low for a minute or two (until totally creamy). You may have to add water for the texture to be correct, but don't forget to take into account the vinegar, oil, and lemon juice. Adjust the seasoning by adding the remaining mix and blending and tasting.

Pour into a serving bowl and drizzle with some more olive oil and tahina mixed with water and salt, if you like, and garnish with red pepper or paprika and a sprig of parsley.

Baked Apples

6 apples

½ cup raisins

¼ cup chopped walnuts

1 tsp. ground cinnamon

1½ cups no-sugar-added apple juice

Wash and core apples; remove peel from around the top. Place apples in 9-inch-square baking dish. Combine raisins, nuts, and cinnamon in small bowl; fill center of each apple with raisin mixture. Pour juice around apples; cover loosely with foil. Bake for 30 to 35 minutes; uncover. Bake for an additional 10 minutes or until tender.

No Wheat, No Dairy, Low Salt

Finding good recipes with no wheat or dairy and low salt can be a challenge. Here are some tasty options.

Orange Zest and Rice

2 cups water

1 tsp. canola oil

1 cup brown rice

1 tsp. orange zest

1 orange, peeled and chopped

¼ cup slivered almonds

Salt and pepper to taste

Bring water to a boil in a heavy saucepan over high heat. Stir in oil, rice, and orange zest and return to a boil. Immediately reduce heat to low. Cover saucepan and simmer 45 minutes or until rice is tender and liquid is absorbed. Remove from heat and set aside 10 minutes. Stir in almonds, salt, and pepper.

Scallop Kabobs

3 medium green peppers, cut into 1½-inch squares

1½ lb. fresh bay scallops

1 pint cherry tomatoes

¼ cup dry white wine

¼ cup vegetable oil

3 TB. lemon juice

Dash garlic powder

Black pepper to taste

Parboil green peppers for 2 minutes. Alternately thread peppers, scallops, and tomatoes on skewers.

Combine wine, oil, lemon juice, garlic powder, and pepper. Brush kabobs with wine mixture, then place on grill (or under broiler). Grill for 15 minutes, turning and basting frequently.

The Least You Need to Know

◆ When following a weight-loss plan, make sure that it's compatible with the anti-inflammation diet.

◆ To reduce hypertension, follow the DASH eating plan, keeping in mind our seven principles.

◆ Look out for hidden sources of gluten or lactose if you are sensitive to either of them.

Appendix A

Glossary

acne   An inflammatory disorder of the skin's oil glands and the areas where hair grows.

aerobic   Involving or improving oxygen consumption by the body, aerobic exercise.

age-related macular degeneration (AMD)   An eye disease that affects the macula, a part of the retina that allows people to see fine detail.

allergy   Inappropriate or exaggerated reactions of the immune system to substances that, in the majority of people, cause no symptoms.

Alzheimer's disease   A progressive brain disease that gradually destroys a person's memory and ability to learn, reason, make judgments, communicate, and carry out daily activities.

amaranth   A grain with a high level of complete protein.

anaphylaxis   A severe, life-threatening allergic reaction.

antioxidant   Any substance that reduces damage due to oxygen (oxidative damage) such as that caused by free radicals.

arachidonic acid (AA)   An omega-6 fatty acid.

arteries   The blood vessels that carry oxygen-rich blood to tissues in your body.

arteriosclerosis   A chronic disease in which thickening, hardening, and loss of elasticity of the arterial walls result in impaired blood circulation.

arthritis   Diseases that generally involve inflammation of the joints. There are more than 100 types.

atherosclerosis   A form of arteriosclerosis characterized by plaques on the inner-most layer of the walls of arteries.

autoimmune diseases   One of a group of diseases, such as rheumatoid arthritis and systemic lupus erythematosus, in which the immune system is overactive and has lost the ability to distinguish between self and non-self.

barley   One of the oldest cultivated grains.

biofeedback   Use of devices that measure such functions as heart rate, body temperature, and muscle tension.

bran   The outer covering of grain.

bromelian   An enzyme from the stem of the pineapple sometimes used to treat pain.

brown rice   Rice that has only the outer hull removed.

buckwheat   The edible fruits of an annual Asian plant used either whole or ground into flour.

bulgur   A quick-cooking form of whole wheat, which has been cleaned, parboiled, dried, ground into particles, and sifted into distinct sizes.

bupleurum   A medicinal root found in East Asia.

cancer   The general name for hundreds of diseases in which some of the body's cells become abnormal and divide without control.

canola oil   A bland monounsaturated oil made from rapeseeds.

carotenoids   The pigments that give fruits and vegetables their bright colors.

cartilage   A firm, rubbery material that covers and protects the ends of bones in normal joints.

cat's claw   An herb that grows in South America.

cayenne   A plant bearing very hot and finely tapering long peppers; usually red.

celiac disease   An immune problem that occurs in response to a protein (gluten) found in all wheat, rye, barley, and triticale products.

complete proteins   Proteins that contain all of the amino acids needed for survival.

corn   Any of numerous cultivated forms of widely grown, annual cereal-grass-bearing grains or kernels on large ears.

corticosteroids   Drugs that closely resemble a hormone called cortisol that the body produces naturally. They are often referred to by the shortened term "steroids."

C-reactive protein (CRP)   A protein in the blood whose level rises dramatically during inflammatory processes occurring in the body.

cytotoxic   Of or relating to substances that are poisonous to cells.

degeneration   The deterioration of specific tissues, cells, or organs with impairment or loss of function.

devil's claw   Any of several herbs of the Southwestern United States and Mexico that have edible pods.

diabetes   A disease in which damaging amounts of sugar build up in the blood.

DMSO   A prescription drug and industrial solvent formed as a by-product of wood-pulp processing.

echinacea   The roots, seeds, or other parts of plants of the genus *Echinacea*, used in herbal medicine.

endocrine organs   Parts of the body that secrete chemicals that control body functions.

endosperm   The food supply of seeds.

essential fatty acids   Fatty acids that cannot be synthesized in the body and must be obtained from the diet.

extra-virgin olive oil   Oil that results from the first pressing of olives.

fat substitutes   Replacements for fat that were developed to help people lower their fat intake.

feverfew   A plant whose leaves are a popular remedy for headaches and migraine.

fiber   A carbohydrate that cannot be digested.

flax   A widely cultivated plant, with seeds that yield linseed oil, and slender stems from which a textile fiber is obtained.

flaxseed oil   Oil obtained from the seeds of the flax plant.

free radicals   Highly reactive chemicals that change chemical structures.

germ   Embryo of the seed, which can sprout into a new plant.

ginger   A tropical plant. The stem of this plant is often used as a spice and to relieve nausea. Also called *gingerroot*.

ginseng   An aromatic root used in traditional Chinese medicine.

glucosamine and chondroitin sulfate   Substances found naturally in the body. Glucosamine is a form of amino sugar that is believed to play a role in cartilage formation and repair. Chondroitin sulfate is part of a large protein molecule (proteoglycan) that gives cartilage elasticity.

gluten   A protein found in wheat or related grains and many foods that we eat. Gluten can be found in a large variety of foods including soups, salad dressings, processed foods and natural flavorings. Unidentified starch, and binders and fillers in medications or vitamins can be unsuspected sources of gluten.

gout   Buildup in the body of too much uric acid, which forms crystals in the joints and causes inflammation.

guggul   A resin from a relative of the myrrh tree, sometimes used to fight pain resulting from inflammation.

heart disease   Any medical condition of the heart or the blood vessels supplying it that impairs cardiac functioning.

high-density lipoprotein (HDL)   The "good" cholesterol. High levels are associated with less coronary disease.

high-sensitivity CRP   A test that measures the amount of a certain protein in the blood (C-reactive protein [CRP]), which can indicate acute inflammation.

hormones   Chemical messengers of the body.

hypnosis   A state of mind between waking and sleeping, sometimes used to cope with pain.

immune system   The integrated body system of organs, tissues, cells, and cell products that recognizes harmful organisms or substances and attacks them.

incomplete proteins   Proteins lacking in one or more of the amino acids.

inflammaging   Describes the connection between inflammation and age-related disease.

inflammation   The body's reaction to injury or to other irritations and stresses such as infections, allergies, chemical irritations, and sometimes loss of function. Common reactions are pain, swelling, redness, and heat. Any area of the body may become inflamed.

inflammatory bowel disease   The general name for diseases that cause inflammation in the intestines. Usually, this refers to Crohn's disease or ulcerative colitis.

insulin   A hormone that is needed to convert sugar, starches, and other food into energy.

itis   A Greek term that means inflammation. For example, colitis is literally inflammation of the colon.

kosher   Conforming to Jewish dietary laws; selling or serving food prepared in accordance with dietary laws.

lactose intolerance   Lactose intolerance is the inability to digest lactose, a type of sugar found in milk and other dairy products. It is caused by a deficiency of the enzyme lactase.

low-density lipoprotein (LDL)   The cholesterol in low-density lipoproteins; the "bad" cholesterol.

licorice   The dried black root of a perennial plant or an extract made from it. It is sought out for possible medicinal qualities.

lycopene   A carotenoid that may reduce the risk of prostate cancer.

macronutrients   The nutrients required in large amounts for normal growth and development. Food has three types of macronutrients: carbohydrate, protein, and fat.

meadowsweet   A perennial herb that grows in damp meadows, sometimes used as a digestive remedy.

meditation   A devotional exercise of or leading to contemplation.

metabolic syndrome   A disorder of metabolism caused by obesity.

metabolism   The series of processes by which food is converted into the energy and products needed to sustain life.

millet   A fast-growing cereal plant that does not have gluten.

monounsaturated fats   Fatty acids that are not "saturated" with hydrogen. They are typically liquid at room temperature, but solidify when refrigerated.

Methylsulfonylmethane (MSM)   A sulfur compound found in the human body.

NSAIDS (non-steroidal anti-inflammatory drugs)   Medications that help control many inflammatory diseases and are used as common over-the-counter pain relievers (examples are ibuprofen [Aleve, Advil], naproxen, etc.).

nut oils   The oils extracted from nuts and low in saturated fats.

obesity   The condition of having an abnormally high proportion of body fat.

olive oil   A blend of virgin oil and refined virgin oil.

olive-pomace oil   A blend of refined olive-pomace oil and virgin oil.

omega-6 fatty acids   Fatty acids that make hormones that lead to inflammation.

omega-3 fatty acids   Fatty acids that make hormones that control inflammation.

osteoarthritis   A type of arthritis that is caused by the breakdown and eventual loss of the cartilage of one or more joints.

overweight   An excess of body weight compared to guidelines set by the Centers for Disease Control.

partially hydrogenated fat   Saturated-like fats made from plant oils and fats.

PCB (polychlorinated biphenyl)   Chemicals used in industrial processes.

phytochemical   A natural compound found in plant foods.

phytoestrogens   Biological agents similar to the hormone estrogen.

plaques   Deposits of fatty material on the inner lining of artery walls.

polymyalgia rheumatica (PMR)   A common cause of aching and stiffness in older adults.

polyunsaturated fats   Fats that are liquid at room temperature, and remain in liquid form even when refrigerated or frozen. They are divided into two families: the omega-3 fats and the omega-6 fats.

processed foods   Foods that have had their shelf life extended through additives.

quinoa   Botanically, a vegetable used as a grain; a complete protein.

refined foods   Highly processed foods.

rheumatoid arthritis   A disease characterized by inflammation of the membranes lining the joints.

rice   An easily digested, widely used grain.

SAM-e   An amino acid derivative that is sometimes used to treat inflammatory conditions.

saturated fat   A fat, most often of animal origin, that is solid at room temperature.

sorghum   A gluten-free grain.

soy protein isolate   A dry powder food ingredient that is made from defatted soy meal.

spelt   A wheat species that is higher in protein than common wheat.

statins   Drugs that stop the body from making too much cholesterol and increase the liver's ability to remove it from blood.

stroke   A condition where brain cells are deprived of blood and stop functioning. Also known as a "brain attack."

tai chi   A Chinese form of physical exercises designed especially for self-defense and meditation.

tempeh   A solid food made by the controlled fermentation of cooked soybeans.

texturized vegetable protein (TVP)   A protein that has been taken from soybeans.

tofu   Also known as soybean curd, a soft food made by curdling fresh hot soy milk with a coagulant.

trans fatty acids   Fats resulting from turning liquid vegetable oil into a solid.

trigger foods   Foods that cause an allergic reaction.

triglycerides   The major form of fat. A triglyceride consists of three molecules of fatty acid combined with a molecule of the alcohol glycerol. Triglycerides serve as the backbone of many types of lipids (fats). Triglycerides come from the food we eat as well as from being produced by the body.

triticale   A new grain that is a hybrid of durum wheat and rye.

unsaturated fat   A fat of plant origin that is liquid at room temperature.

vegan   A vegetarian who eats only plant products.

vegetarian   One who eats primarily fruits and vegetables and vegetable products.

virgin olive   Fine extra-virgin and virgin olive oils are processed through cold or mechanical pressing. This is a natural, chemical-free process involving only pressure, which produces a low level of acidity in the oil.

visualization   The use of imagery to focus the mind.

walnut oil   Oil extracted from walnuts and rich in omega-3 fatty acids.

wheat   A grain that contains large amounts of gluten, which causes baked goods to rise.

whole grains   The edible intact seeds of plants.

wild rice   The seed of an aquatic grass.

willow bark   Bark of the willow tree, used throughout the centuries in China and Europe to treat fever, pain, headache, and inflammatory conditions such as arthritis.

yoga   A Hindu discipline aimed at training the consciousness for a state of perfect spiritual insight and tranquility.

Resources

Health Organizations

Alzheimer's Association
225 N. Michigan Ave., Fl. 17
Chicago, IL 60601-7633
1-800-272-3900
www.alz.org

American Academy of Allergy, Asthma & Immunology
555 E. Wells St.
Suite 1100
Milwaukee, WI 53202-3823
414-272-6071 or 1-800-822-2762
www.aaaai.org

American Autoimmune and Related Diseases Association
National Office
22100 Gratiot Ave.
East Detroit, MI 48021
586-776-3900
www.aarda.org

American Cancer Society
(Call for location of local chapter)
1-800-ACS-2345 or 1-866-228-4327 (TTY)
www.cancer.org

American College of Allergy, Asthma & Immunology
85 West Algonquin Rd., Suite 550
Arlington Heights, IL 60005
www.acaai.org

The American College of Cardiology
Heart House
9111 Old Georgetown Road
Bethesda, MD 20814-1699
1-800-253-4636, ext. 694 or 301-897-5400
Fax: 301-897-9745
www.acc.org

American Diabetes Association
1701 N. Beauregard St.
Alexandria, VA 22311
1-800-DIABETES (1-800-342-2383)
www.diabetes.org

American Heart Association
National Center
7272 Greenville Ave.
Dallas, TX 75231
1-800-AHA-USA-1 (1-800-242-8721)
www.americanheart.org

American Sleep Apnea Association
1424 K Street NW, Suite 302
Washington, D.C. 20005
202-293-3650
Fax: 202-293-3656
www.sleepapnea.org

Arthritis Foundation
P.O. Box 7669
Atlanta, GA 30357-0669
404-872-7100 or 1-800-568-4045
www.arthritis.org

Asthma and Allergy Foundation of America
1233 20th St. NW
Suite 402
Washington, D.C. 20036
1-800-7ASTHMA (1-800-727-8462)
www.aafa.org

Celiac Disease Foundation
13251 Ventura Blvd., #1
Studio City, CA 91604
818-990-2354 or 818-990-2379
www.celiac.org

Center for Science in the Public Interest
1875 Connecticut Ave. N.W.
Suite 300
Washington, D.C. 20009
202-332-9110
cspi@cspinet.org

Centre for Science in the Public Interest
Suite 4550, CTTC Bldg.
1125 Colonel By Dr.
Ottawa, Ontario K1S 5R1
Canada
613-244-7337
jefferyb@istar.ca

The Food Allergy & Anaphylaxis Network
11781 Lee Jackson Hwy., Suite 160
Fairfax, VA 22033-3309
703-691-2713 or 1-800-929-4040
www.foodallergy.org

Macular Degeneration Foundation, Inc.
P.O. Box 531313
Henderson, NV 89053
1-888-633-3937
www.eyesight.org

National Stroke Association
9707 E. Easter Lane
Englewood, CO 80112
National Stroke Association
1-800-STROKES (1-800-787-6537)

Oldways Preservation Trust
266 Beacon St.
Boston, MA 02116
617-421-5500
oldways@oldwayspt.org

Organic Foods

Alternative Farming Systems Information Center
10301 Baltimore Ave., Room 132
Beltsville, MD 20705-2351
301-504-6559
TDD: 301-504-6856
Fax: 301-504-6409
afsic@nal.usda.gov

FoodRoutes
37 East Durham Street
Philadelphia, PA 19119
814-349-6000
www.foodroutes.org

Just Food
208 East 51st Street, 4th Floor
New York, NY 10022
212-645-9880
Fax: 212-645-9881
www.justfood.org

LocalHarvest
220 21st Ave.
Santa Cruz, CA 95062
831-475-8150
Fax: 831-401-2418
www.localharvest.org/contact.jsp

National Cooperative Grocers Association
1104 Weeber Circle
Iowa City, IA 52246
319-466-9029
www.cooperativegrocer.coop

Organic Consumers Association
6771 South Silver Hill Drive
Finland, MN 55603
218-226-4164
Fax: 218-353-7652
www.organicconsumers.org/

Slow Food
International office:
Via Mendicità Istruita, 8
12042 Bra (CN) Italy

+39 0172 419 611
Fax: +39 0172 421293
international@slowfood.com

USA office:
info@slowfoodusa.org
20 Jay Street #313, Brooklyn, NYC
NY 10013 USA
718-260-8000 or 1-718-260-8068

U.S. Government Agencies

Administration on Aging
330 Independence Ave. SW
Washington, D.C. 20201
1-202-619-7501

Centers for Disease Control and Prevention
1600 Clifton Rd.
Atlanta, GA 30333
404-639-3534 or 1-800-311-3435

Eldercare Locator
1-800-677-1116
www.eldercare.gov

National Asthma Education and Prevention Program
NHLBI Health Information Network
P.O. Box 30105
Bethesda, MD 20824-0105
301-592-8573
Fax: 301-592-8563
www.nhlbi.nih.gov

National Heart Attack Alert Program
NHLBI Health Information Network
P.O. Box 30105
Bethesda, MD 20824-0105
301-592-8573
Fax: 301-592-8563
www.nhlbi.nih.gov

National Heart, Lung, and
Blood Institute
P.O. Box 30105
Bethesda, MD 20824-0105
301-592-8573 or 240-629-3255 (TTY)
www.nhlbi.nih.gov

USDA Food and Nutrition
Information Center (FNIC)
10301 Baltimore Ave., Room 304
Beltsville, MD 20705-2351
301-504-5719
www.nal.usda.gov/fnic

U.S. Food and Drug Administration
5600 Fishers Lane
Rockville, MD 20857-0001
1-888-INFO-FDA (1-888-463-6332)

Canadian Government Agencies

Public Health Agency of Canada
130 Colonnade Rd.
A.L. 6501H
Ottawa, Ontario K1A 0K9
www.phac-aspc.gc.ca/new_e.html

Public Health Agency of Canada
1015 Arlington St.
Winnipeg, Manitoba R3E 3R2
www.phac-aspc.gc.ca/new_e.html

Websites and Publications

The following websites and publications provide additional information on anti-inflammation, including where to go for help and nutritional information.

Websites

Consumer Health Websites

American Cancer Society
Calculates your daily calorie needs.
www.cancer.org/docroot/PED/content/PED_6_1x_Calorie_Calculator.asp

Canadian Health Network (CHN)
Offers FAQs and articles on health from Health Canada, organized by topic and by group.
www.canadian-health-network.ca

CRP Health
Information on C-reactive protein for professionals and consumers.
www.crphealth.com/home/gen

FamilyDoctor
Health information for the whole family from the American Academy of Family Physicians.
www.familydoctor.org

Federal Agencies

The federal government has several websites with information on nutrition:

- www.nutrition.gov
- www.healthierus.gov
- www.mypyramid.gov

Health.gov
List of U.S. government sites related to health issues and topics.
www.health.gov

Intelihealth
Comprehensive collection of consumer health information.
www.intelihealth.com

Mayo Clinic
Offers information on diseases and conditions, healthy living, drugs, and self-care.
www.mayoclinic.com

Medscape
A comprehensive online search service from WebMD. Provides health and medical information.
www.medscape.com

MSN Health & Fitness
This interactive tool measures how many calories are burned during many common activities.
www.health.msn.com/dietnutrition/articlepage.aspx?cp-documentid=100106088

My Pyramid
Guide to the Food and Drug Administration's 2005 food pyramid.
www.mypyramid.gov

National Center for Health Statistics
BMI charts for children.
www.cdc.gov/growthcharts

WebMD
Features a wide range of medical information, health and wellness tips, and health news.
www.webmd.com

Nutrition Websites

American Dietetic Association (ADA)
Contains nutritional information and resources. Also offers a directory of dietitians.
www.eatright.org

Fast Food Facts
Nutritional information on fast foods.
www.foodfacts.info

Glycemic Index
This is the website for the glycemic index and international GI database which is based at the University of Sydney.
www.glycemicindex.com

Healthier Fast Food Choices
Nutritional data for the healthier fast foods.
www.healthchecksystems.com/ffood.htm

Nutrient Data Laboratory
Lists nutritional values of foods.
www.ars.usda.gov/nutrientdata

NutritionData
Nutrient analysis for any food or recipe.
www.nutritiondata.com

Oldways Preservation Trust
Aims to help consumers make wise food choices.
www.oldwayspt.org

Organic Kitchens
Web's gateway to information about organic food.
www.organickitchen.com

Whole Grains Council
Online guide to whole grains.
www.wholegrainscouncil.org

Publications

Magazines and Newsletters

Consumer Reports on Health
Online newsletter
www.consumerreports.org/main/crh/home.jsp

Food Reflections Newsletter
University of Nebraska Cooperative Extension
Free e-mail subscription
www.lancaster.unl.edu/food/foodtalk.htm

Nutrition Action Health Letter
U.S. mailing address:
Center for Science in the Public Interest
1875 Connecticut Ave. NW
Suite 300
Washington, D.C. 20009
202-332-9110
cspi@cspinet.org

Canadian mailing address:
Centre for Science in the Public Interest
Suite 4550, CTTC Bldg.
1125 Colonel By Drive
Ottawa, Ontario K1S 5R1
Canada
613-244-7337
jefferyb@istar.ca

Tufts University Health & Nutrition Letter
Subscription Department
P.O. Box 420235
Palm Coast, FL 32142-0235
1-800-274-7581
www.healthletter.tufts.edu/contact.html

Books

Critser, Greg. *Fat Land: How Americans Became the Fattest People in the World.* New York: Houghton Mifflin, 2003.

Nestle, Marion. *Food Politics: How the Food Industry Influences Nutrition and Health.* Berkeley, CA: University of California Press, 2002.

Schlosser, Eric. *Fast Food Nation: The Dark Side of the All-American Meal.* New York: Harper Perennial, 2001.

Willett, Walter C. *Eat, Drink, and Be Healthy: The Harvard Medical School Guide to Healthy Eating.* New York: Free Press, 2005.

Cookbooks

American Heart Association. *The New American Heart Association Cookbook.* New York: Ballantine, 2001.

Berry, Barbara. *5 a Day: The Better Health Cookbook; Savor the Flavor of Fruits and Vegetables.* Emmaus, PA: Rodale, 2002.

The Food Allergy & Anaphylaxis Network. *The Food Allergy News Cookbook: A Collection of Recipes from Food Allergy News and Members of the Food Allergy Network.* New York: John Wiley & Sons, Inc., 1998.

Gass, Gerald, Maren Caruso, Nan McEvoy, Joyce Goldstein, and Jacqueline Mallorca. *The Olive Harvest Cookbook: Olive Oil Lore and Recipes from McEvoy Ranch.* San Francisco, CA: Chronicle, 2004.

Hensrud, Donald D., Jennifer Nelson, Cheryl Forberg, Maureen Callahan, and Sheri Giblin. *The New Mayo Clinic Cookbook: Eating Well for Better Health.* Birmingham, AL: Oxmoor House, 2004.

Reinhardt-Martin, Jane. *The Amazing Flax Cookbook.* Washington, D.C.: TSA Press, 2004.

Yarnell, Elizabeth. *Glorious One-Pot Meals.* Denver, CO: Pomegranate Consulting, 2005.

Index